The Crucible: And the Firs

© 2010   The Crucible: And the Fires of Chang
          L. Michael Hall, Ph.D.

Library of Congress, Washington, D.C.
Copyright Pending
ISBN: 9781890001384

All rights reserved.
No part of this may be reproduced, stored in a retrieval system, or transmitted in any form or by any means (electronic, mechanical, photocopying, recording, etc.) without the prior written permission of the publisher.

Published by: NSP —*Neuro-Semantics Publications*
                     P.O. Box 8
                     Clifton, CO. 81520-0008 USA
                     (970) 523-7877

Neuro-Semantics® is the trademark name for the models, patterns, and society of Neuro-Semantics. ISNS is the initials of the International Society of Neuro-Semantics— a world-wide network of trainers, coaches, and consultants committed to *Actualizing Excellence* within individuals and organizations. For more than 4000 pages of free information, see the web sites:
          www.neurosemantics.com
          www.meta-coaching.org
          www.self-actualizing.org
          www.nlp-video.com

Acknowledgment:
Sue Anderson, Australia, a Meta-Coach provided much of the proof-reading for this text.

THE CRUCIBLE — CONTENTS

Preface:
The Magic of the Crucible   1

Part I: A Crucible for Human Energies   7

1. *The Crucible Matrix*   8
   Tested and Tried for Self-Actualization

2. *Changed for Good!*   19
   Two models of Change for Unleashing Your Highest and Best

3. *Crucibles: An Encounter with Reality*   29

4. *Why the Crucible Model?*   39
   Crucible Benefits and Elements

5. *The Crucible and Emotions*   55
   Transforming Emotions

6. *Everyday Crucibles*   68
   Using Life's Challenges, traumas and disappointments as Crucibles

Part II: Crucible Elements   79
7. *Unconditional Positive Regard*

8. *Witnessing*   96
   Pure Attention of What *Is*

9. *Acceptance*   109
   The Magic of acknowledgment

10. *The Truth*   120
    The Heart of Authenticity

11. *Appreciation*   137
    The Sacrilizing Art

12. *Responsibility*   147
    The Power of Response

13. *Joyous Love*   163
    Peaking Out of the Crucible

Part III: Transformation in the Crucible   169
14. *The Crucible Trance*   170
    Patterns for Entering the Crucible

15. *The Crucible Conversation*   182
    Fierce center at the heart of things

16. *The Crucible and Coaching*   190

Appendices   195
Appendix A: Cognitive Distortions
Appendix B: Meta-Coaching   196

Bibliography   197

Index   200

Author   202

PREFACE

The Magic of the Crucible

What is the Crucible?
The Crucible is a space for transformational change so you can actualize your highest and best. It is a wonderful hypnotic space you create within your mind for generative change. It is a model for unlearning (as well as learning) and for a deep personal encounter with yourself.

The Crucible is not a real place in the outside world; it is a real place in the inside world of your mind—if you create it there. This book is your personal invitation to create a powerful place in your mind — a place where the magic of transformation can happen. This book is my invitation to you to create a place where you can facilitate change that will occur easily, naturally, and organically. With this process you can invent a place where you can break through your old defenses and foolishness, even your old B.S. that has undermined your genius and glory for all these years. Would you like to do that?

The Crucible, as an incredible hypnotic induction, is designed for your authenticity. It is designed as a change place for you to actualize your highest values and visions in your best performances. Are you ready for ecstasy? Are you ready to fall in love with life, with the adventure of discovery and growth? Are you ready for the vitality of being fully alive/fully human? If so, buy this book, read it, absorb it, use it to be coached to your next-level of development. If not, put it down immediately and run as fast as you can! If not, this book will be dangerous to your "peace of mind."

The metaphor of a Crucible, as used here as a picture of change and transformation, arises from two sources—industry and artists. In both cases, a crucible is used to melt down iron ore and other elements which can then be poured into molds that give the metal new form and strength. The crucible is the holding space for all of this transformation of molten materials.

Who is *The Crucible* for?
As a book on self-actualization, *The Crucible* is a book of processes that trainers, coaches, leaders, managers, parents, and anyone else can use. If you want to facilitate *the self-actualizing process* and enable yourself and others to unleash latent potentials—this book is for you. Yet it is more than just processes for development. As a place for self-actualizing transformation, the Crucible enables you to create and enter a sacred space that protects and honors human possibilities and transcendence.

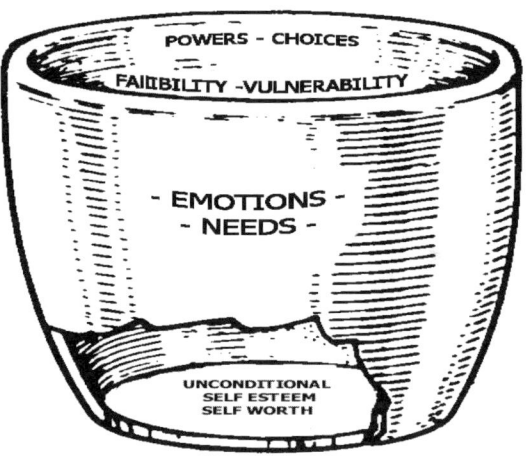

In this book you will learn the process for how to create a Crucible space for yourself and for another. To illustrate this, I have provided numerous case studies of those who have entered the Crucible for a metamorphosis of old habits, limiting beliefs, and sabotaging understandings. In this pages I will also tell the story of how this process developed the Crucible as a pattern and a model.

Where is the book *The Crucible* Positioned?
The Crucible is the seventh book in the *Meta-Coaching* book series. As such it presents the second change model of Meta-Coaching. You'll learn all about this in chapter two where I'll explain the Crucible as a change model and compare it to *The Axes of Change Model* that is fully described in Meta-Coaching Volume I.

This is also the fourth book in the series on Self-Actualization and Self-Actualization Psychology which is the psychology for the emergent field of Coaching. Why? Because unlike therapy, Coaching works primarily with people who are psychologically healthy and who are ready to get on with the highest challenges in the adventure of life.

Where did the Idea and Elements of *The Crucible* come from?
It came from the developers of the first Human Potential Movement (HPM) of the 1960s. I found almost all of the pieces for the construction of the Crucible in the writings of Abraham Maslow, Carl Rogers, Rollo May, Robert Assagioli and other leaders of the first Human Potential Movement. They had an intuitive sense that people would self-actualize if they had *a personal "encounter" with the truth of their life experiences and the truth of their own meaning-making.* Via that encounter a person becomes real and authentic which then empowers them to translate what is potential into actuality. In other words, I didn't invent this from scratch, I found it and put it together in the form that follows.

Why was that Inadequate?
Now several of these original thinkers of the HPM did put together many of the Crucible pieces. But they did not put enough of them together. Now some of them thought they did! Some of them even argued that what they put together was fully sufficient to facilitate self-actualization. It was not. For example, Carl Rogers presented his now famous three-fold recommendation of the qualities that he considered "necessary and sufficient for healing and self-actualizing." He thought unconditional positive regard, accurate empathy, and personal congruency or authenticity were enough. And he was close, very close, and yet there were still a few things missing from that formulation. I'll describe this more fully in chapter 10 on "Truth."

Did the Leaders of the first HPM Discover the Secret?
Well, yes, they discovered many of the secrets! Yet not one of them put all of the elements together. They knew that there had to be an intense, focused, and life-changing *encounter* and they worked to create it, but the kind of "encounter" prevalent among the people of that first movement was not adequate for the consistent unleashing of potentials.

And why not? Primarily because the Encounter Groups at those early years were too brutal, confrontative, too rough, and too threatening, and so evoked as much fear and defensiveness as it did hope and transformative vision. It was an undependable process. So those Encounter Groups eventually faded away. And the primary reason for that was singular—*there wasn't sufficient safety in the encounter.* There wasn't sufficient reduction of the danger and so the basic human defense mechanisms were never sufficiently calmed.

Standing on their Shoulders, What has been Learned?
Today we know something that they didn't know, namely, that the releasing of potentials doesn't have to be rough or explicitly confrontative. We don't have to "get in someone's face" and "break through their defenses" to enable the self-actualization process. Unleashing can occur much more subtly, often by simply the uncovering processes (processes that enable us to uncover that's hidden within).

This is one of the best discoveries of *The Crucible Model* that you will experience in this book. You can now create a space that allows yourself and others to relax defenses, posturing, and hiding behind personas. You can create a space that enables a person to let go of all of the barriers to authenticity because there's no need to personalize the threats. And by eliminating the tendency to personalize, you eliminate the need to defend yourself—as if it needed defending.

While the first human potential movement was on the right track, they didn't quite get the self-actualization formula right. But now, these many decades later, we are able to see things they didn't. This has nothing to do with a superior intellect or skill. We see further than they did because we stand on their shoulders. Today we have learned from their insights and contributions as well as mistakes and mis-applications. Here I have made the discoveries explicit and then extended them in new ways.

Is it Possible to Create a Safe, Loving Encounter?
Yes! *The Crucible Model* enables you to have an encounter with truth, with the truths you need to face, and the truths that will set you free to be yourself fully and authentically. The Crucible creates the safety so that you can do that without personalizing and without feeling threatened. *And here's another fascinating discovery—you can even do this with yourself.*

Then, once you enter the center sanctum of the Crucible, you not only face the truth, but you find value in it through "the continual freshness of appreciation" that characterizes self-actualizing people. And that, in turn, then enables you to take full ownership and responsibility of your insights, realizations, and discoveries thereby altering your character forever.

By iterating that process you will then move up the levels of authenticity, the levels of truth, and the levels of appreciation and responsibility. Then suddenly, unexpectedly, surprisingly you'll experience a "peak experience." Ah, the peak experience! That's when love and joy breaks in to surprise you. And these emotions serve as signs and indicators that you have entered into the zone of self-actualization and that you are transcending yourself.

What do you mean *The Crucible* is Hypnotic?
Ah yes, hypnotic, hypnosis, trance, the inner world, the magic of representation and meaning and frames! The boy potential mysteriously said to Neo in the movie, *The Matrix,* "There is no spoon..." So also *there is no Crucible.* There are only your constructed images and memories and imaginations and feelings and beliefs and intentions and hopes and dreams that come together to create a place for transformative change— in your mind, in your heart. "Think not that it is the spoon that moves; it is rather you who moves."

Hypnosis!? Yes and no. As it is inside you, and as it is created by you, you have to *transition* from the outside state of sights, sounds, and sensations to your inside state of sights, sounds, and sensations. And it is that inside state that we call *trance* since you transitioned there and when you are there, you seem to be gone, lost, not present to the outside world. So centuries ago, people called that "sleep" or hypnosis. But you are not really asleep, you are just *inside*— fully awake to your possibilities!

And being inside—*fully awake to yourself and your highest objectives*—you are now free and empowered to build up a resource within so that you can adapt, change, unlearn, and actualize your highest and best potentials.

What Else is in *The Crucible?*
You will find that each chapter ends with an invitation for some *Crucible Coaching.* Would you like that? I hope so. If I were with you in person and had the opportunity to encourage you to integrate and implement what you just read, I would coach you to your next-level step of self-actualizing. Since I'm not there in person, I have provided some *Crucible Coaching* to complete each chapter.

If you want to really take advantage of that, get a notebook and title it, *My Transformational Life.* Then as you complete each chapter, use the coaching paragraphs to apply and implement what you've learned so that it becomes actualized performance in your life. This will raise the value of the book to giving you a three-thousand dollar value for your money.

I've included in this book many *Self-Actualizing Patterns*, especially in the Elements of the Crucible chapters. From the field of Neuro-Semantics, now you can build up your hypnotic transformational breakthrough space by using these processes for actualizing your ability to change with graceful power.

I'm delighted to send forth this book about this incredibly powerful and gentle process under the provocative title— *The Crucible*. My hope is that this will empower coaches, consultants, trainers, leaders, and everybody who works with people to facilitate the unleashing of human potentials in hundreds of thousands. I trust that this will enable people everywhere to find their own authenticity and live their integrity congruently. I hope also that many will use *the Crucible process* for creating new metamorphosis for themselves transforming old structures of beliefs, habits, decisions, understandings, etc. into new empowering and enlivening ones.

So with that in mind, here's to your transformative changes that will make you feel incredibly more alive, more human, and more able to live your potentials!

L. Michael Hall, Ph.D.
Colorado, 2010

Part I

A Crucible

For

Human Energies

Chapter 1

THE CRUCIBLE MATRIX

Tested and Tried for Self-Actualization

Why a Crucible? Why would you need such a thing? *For self-actualization of course!* Why else? The one and only purpose of the Crucible is to facilitate you finding, tapping into, unleashing, releasing, and developing your highest visions and values and living your best performances. In that light, *the Crucible is a tool* (or human technology) *enabling you to create the best version of you.*

Now as we begin, I want to issue a warning: This will not be easy or fast. If unleashing and actualizing your highest and best human potentials were easy, everybody would be living on the cutting-edge of life and producing peak performances! If it were easy and fast, everybody would be pushing themselves to the height of their possibilities. Everybody would be experiencing lots of peak experiences in everyday life, living in ecstasy, and transforming their best activities into peak performances. If it was easy and fast, everybody you know would be feeling the ecstasy of giving their all and expressing the full range of their uniqueness. But, sadly, it is not. It is not easy. Nor is it fast.

In fact, this will demand everything of you—it will demand all of you. There will be times when you will find it extremely challenging. So are you still game? Actualizing your highest and best is one of the most demanding experiences for a human being. And that's why most of us are not unleashing our potentials in service of actualizing our self and our greatest potentials. It does require a complete commitment to your possibilities.

Now if that is the bad news, here's the good news. Paradoxically and ironically, *you, like all of us, are driven and motivated for self-actualization.* It is one of our highest drives. All of you have this drive. It drives you from the inside just as much as the purely biological drives for air, food, water, and shelter. It drives you just as much as the bio-social drives for safety, friendship, and love and affection. And it drives you just as much as your bio-psychological drives for self-regard, self-worth, self-importance, and dignity. It is one of your higher needs and one at a qualitatively higher level.

The problem with this drive, if we can rightly call it a "problem," is that *it requires consciousness.* You have to mindfully choose to give yourself to this drive. Otherwise, you will avoid it, deny it, escape it, defend against it, fear it, hate it, and so on. This means that you have to participate not only in detecting this drive, but welcoming it into your consciousness. You have to assume responsibility for it, and have to expend effort to actualize it. Are you willing to do all of that?

Fulfilling this drive of self-actualization is not an absolute requirement for life. To experience this level of vitality you have to cooperate with the drive, cultivate it, and choose it. You can live without it. Yet after you satisfy the other drives, you cannot thrive or live a purposefully meaningful life without responding to it. This is a drive that requires and involves your spirit, your sense of purpose and transcendence. This also describes the nature of self-actualization, namely, that you have to be *awakened* to it—much as Neo was.

It's Like Neo in "The Matrix Movie"
Unleashing your highest potentials within the Crucible is not unlike what Neo went through in the Matrix Movie. So I'll use that as an illustration.[1]

Have you seen the movie? If not, the central hero is Neo (the new one) who was awakened to the Matrix. That began the adventure. He then made the decision to take the red pill and escape the Matrix. Later he re-entered the Matrix. That allowed him to learn its rules and become trained in mastering the Matrix. By re-entering it he discovered how he could fight "the system of control" and become *the One,* foretold by the Oracle, who would master the Matrix.

In this, Neo followed his self-actualization drive and entered a number of crucibles, all of which enabled him to unleash the potentials awaiting to be unleashed. In the movie, Neo was enslaved to "the Matrix" but didn't even know it. The Matrix *had* him, but he was unaware of that fact or even that there was such a thing as a matrix.

So the first movie opened with him slowly becoming aware of "the matrix." Then as he became increasingly awakened to the Matrix, he had to make a decision. Would he take the red pill and escape the Matrix or would he take the blue pill and stay in it, believing whatever he wanted to believe, and live oblivious to the nature of that world? He took the red pill. After he recovered from the ordeal, he was invited to re-enter the Construct of the Matrix to learn its rules and to become trained in the art of mastering the Matrix. Through that matrix training, he was then able to re-enter the Matrix to fight the "system of control" of the Matrix and its agents. And in that way, he could actualize the vision that Morpheus had awakened in him of becoming *the One* who would master the Matrix.

This story, as it turns out, is not all that far or different from the actual conditions of our lives. We too live in a Matrix —a matrix of meaning and belief frames about the world. We also were born into that Matrix—a matrix constructed by those who came before us, those in our immediate blood family and those who created our language, our history, our culture. It is made up of our individual family cultural frames, religious frames, the linguistic frames inherent in our language, in the frames of the educational system, government system, and all of the other frames that we were born into.

And like Neo, most of us do not wake up to this realization until many years later. Then we may or may not realize that the Matrix of all of these frames about the meaning of things *has* us. As long as we are blind to it, we are a servant to its frames. Those frames govern how we think and feel, how we perceive things, respond, and experience life itself. And yet, ultimately, *our life experience is a function of the meaning frames we learn and accept.*

Now, of course, as with any metaphor we can only take *The Matrix Movie* so far. After that the metaphor breaks down. So while I use the Matrix Movie as a metaphor, there are numerous places where it does not carry over to our experience as human beings who are born in a Matrix of cultural and family frames and who absorb and create additional meaning frames about things. One facet that does carry over is the experience in the Matrix of being tested and refined as if in a crucible.

The Crucible of Questions and Collaboration
While Neo eventually became *the one*, and was able to master that Matrix as he unleashed his potentials, it was not an easy or fast process. Along the way to his full self-actualization, he went through numerous crucible experiences.

Neo's first crucible experience was with Trinity. She had sent a message on his computer after he fell asleep on his keyboard. "Wake up Neo, the Matrix has you!" Then another, "Follow the White Rabbit." That led Neo to a nightclub where he seemed out of place. That's when Trinity approached him and whispered in his ear:
> "It is the question that drives us, Neo. It is the question that brought you here. You know the question, just as I did. The answer is out there, Neo."

Neo: "What is the Matrix?"

In this encounter, Trinity indicated that the answer to this central question was "out there" and that Neo had to extend himself to begin his exploration to find that answer. And as he was looking for the answer to, "What is the matrix?," so she and Morpheus had been looking for him. And so were the Sentinel Agents; they were also looking for Neo and finding him at work, they arrested him. They also tested his resolve and then sent him away having put a "bug" in him.

The next thing that happened was Trinity's phone call to Neo to set up a rendezvous with Morpheus. Yet because the Agents had bugged Neo, he had to be de-bugged. So, pulling out a terrifying gun-like machine, asked him to pull up his shirt, and put the de-bugging machine on his stomach. It was too much. "Stop the car!" he ordered. Then opening the door, he was ready to bolt into the rain on that dark and gloomy night.
> "You don't want to go down that road Neo. You've been down

that path before, you know where it goes."

All of this was a crucible experience for Neo. In these moments of confusion, threat, insecurity, decision, etc., his spirit and character was being tested. Would he have to do things his way, or would he be able to work with others and become a member of the team of those who were part of the rebellion against the Machines?

The Crucible of Choice
The next crucible occurred in his dialogue with Morpheus when he was confronted with a life-changing choice, the choice between the red and the blue pills.

Morpheus:
> "Let me tell you why you are here. You have come because you know something. What you know you can't explain, but you feel it. You've felt it your whole life, felt that something is wrong with the world. You don't know what, but it's there like a splinter in your mind, driving you mad. It is this feeling that brought you to me. You know what I'm talking about?"

Neo: "The Matrix?"
Morpheus: "Do you want to know what *it* is?"
Neo: "Yes."
Morpheus: "The Matrix is everywhere, it's all around us . . . It is the world that has been pulled down over your eyes to blind you from the truth."
Neo: "The truth?"
Morpheus:
> "That you are a slave, Neo. Like everyone else, you were born into bondage, kept inside a prison that you cannot smell, taste, or touch. A prison for your mind." (Wachowski, 2000, p. 300)
>
> "It seems you're feeling a bit like Alice, tumbling down the rabbit hole. You have the look of a man who accepts what he sees because he is expecting to wake up.
>
> "You were born into slavery, into a prison that you cannot see or smell . . . *A prison of the mind* . . . Unfortunately, no one can tell you what the Matrix is; you have to see it for yourself."

Since "no one can tell you what it is," Morpheus invited Neo to see the Matrix for himself. Presenting two pills, Morpheus held in his hands, a blue one and a red one. This was another test— a test of Neo's will, of his commitment, of his willingness to discover the truth.

> "Take the Blue Pill, and you will wake up in your bed and believe whatever you want to believe. Take the red pill and you stay in Wonder Land, and I'll show you how deep the Rabbit Hole goes."

The Crucible of Being Tested
In *The Matrix* Movie, Neo's most challenging crucible was the constant testing by the Agents as the Sentinels of the Matrix, and especially Mr. Smith. They were everywhere inside the Matrix and yet they did not exist as a single person. That's because, as "programs" designed to search out "anomalies," (i.e., Neo), these Sentinel guards of the Matrix could enter into the form of anyone who's inside the Matrix, anyone still plugged in. This made everyone plugged into the Matrix a potential agent. Even though the humans were imprisoned in egg-like structures so that the energy of their brains could be harvested, they were also having "information" jacked into their nervous system which thereby deceived them regarding where they were and what they were doing.

The weakness and the vulnerability of the Agents is that they were governed by the rules of the Matrix. This meant that they can never be as fast or as strong as *the One who masters the Matrix*. When Morpheus explains this to Neo, Neo's questions were incredulous.

> "You mean I will be faster than a bullet?"

Morpheus' answer seemed vague and yet it foreshadowed what was yet to come. "When you are there, you won't have to be." Yet to unleash that possibility, Neo had many fights with the agents, many chase scenes and many testings of his spirit. These also were his crucibles in the Matrix.

The Crucible of Training Preparation
When Morpheus first took Neo into the Construct, it was to learn—to learn about the Matrix, how it works, its rules, its limits. After Neo learned Kong Fu, a sparring match takes place between Neo and Morpheus because Morpheus wanted to see what he had learned and what he could do. There also, Morpheus defeated Neo, and then commented,

> "Your weakness is not your technique."

He made the comment almost under his breath. Then he asked,
> "Why did I defeat you?"

As Neo was then in quiet reflection, he commented:
> "Do you believe that my being stronger or faster has anything to do with my muscles in this place? You think that's air you're breathing now?"

All of this was designed to awaken Neo's awareness to the reality and nature of the Matrix—*it is just information.* The data being sent to his brain by the machines was hypnotizing and seducing him. And believing it to be real was the way Neo's mind was defeating him. So what does mastering the Matrix mean? It means freeing the mind of false beliefs and understandings and using it powerfully for one's full development.

As they continued the fight to test his skills, Morpheus then said:
> "Stop *trying* to hit me and *hit* me."

Ah, another crucible— one designed to free his mind from the constraints that the frames of that Matrix had presented. And that's what any crucible worth its weight does— it gives us a chance to challenge our assumptions, clearing out limiting beliefs, and seeing the truth for what it is.

The Crucible and Self-Actualization

In the adventure of actualizing your highest and best, you also will go through numerous crucible experiences. More often than not, those who become their best selves, those who tap into their innate potentials for greatness, go through many trying experiences. And to what end? How are challenging experiences useful? Experiences that try your spirit are useful because they put you to the test and enable you to call forth what lies deep within. It tests your metal. It cultivates your spirit and character. It happened to Nelson Mandella, to Martin Luther King Jr., and to many who today we call "great."

Abraham Maslow, the pioneer of Self-Actualization Psychology, noted that it is through capitalizing on tough times that those we recognize as great people became who they became and achieved the heights that they achieved.

> "We should study the psychotherapeutic effects of bad experiences,

particularly of tragedy, but also illness, deprivation, frustration, conflict, and the like. Healthy people seem able to turn even such experiences to good use." (1970, p. 287)

Maslow took this even further. He went so far as to suggest that we can (and should) learn to see *any* and *every* failure to achieve self-actualization as psycho-pathology (1970, p. 286). That is, you and I are not whole, are not healthy, are not what we are designed to be *when we are not actively pursuing our fullest self-actualization.*

After all, that's the purpose of human life—to be your best version of you, to become as fully human and fully alive as possible, and to be true to yourself and the potentials that you have to offer. Anything less is a form of sickness which should not be tolerated. You are not meant just to get by, just to pass the time, or to look busy, you are meant to develop as fully as possible, to experience what you are potentially able to become and to contribute from this inner richness.

So bring on the crucibles! Bring on the experiences of life that test your spirits and refine your character, the experiences that enable you to unleash those potentials that you are just barely awakened to! And let the adventure begin!

Crucibling the Fear of Failure
When I worked with Juan, the subject that he wanted to address was "the fear of failure." When I asked him, "What would trigger that fear?" he began talking about "stepping up to higher responsibilities" as a manager. If he thought about that, then an internal feeling of the fear of failure would become incredibly intense. The synonyms that he used for what he then felt were "anguished, anxiety, depressed and paralysis."

"So give me an example of a challenge that involves higher responsibilities that would elicit that kind of state," I asked him. He talked about almost anything *new* that he was not familiar with, anything that would be a test of his managerial skills, and that could reflect on the success of his career path. I then inquired about how intense this was.

"A '10' on the scale. The fear absolutely paralyzes me; I just freeze. I can't do anything."

"Wow!" I said and paused for effect. "You are so masterful at this fear! Here we are sitting in these comfortable chairs at this Conference Center in this beautiful setting and all you have to do is think about an upcoming event, and boom! You go into paralyzing fear that fast!" I said snapping my fingers. "How do you do that? What mastery!"

"Well..." he paused. "I don't know. It's like a piece of dust in the gears of a machine that then makes the whole machine useless."

"Let me get this straight: one piece of dust— *one*— and then the machinery is useless! [Yes] And you believe this?"

"Yes," he said in the most matter-of-fact way.

"And you're talking about you? One little flaw or mistake or something and *you* are suddenly useless? Is that what you believe?"

"Yes."

"So what, you have to be perfect? You have to be God-like, flawless?"

"Well, you know I have always had this little joke, There are two perfect ones."

"Oh, so now you are running for 'God?' Or maybe you are his best and equal rival? And you believe this?"

"Well I know I make mistakes and that being a human being means being imperfect."

"Stop the presses! Did I just hear the solution? Did you just put the answer to all of this out on the table?"

"Yes, I know that. I know that I need to accept my humanity, but I just can't. When I do it doesn't last, it is just temporary."

"So you need to just *accept* yourself because..."

"Because I am a human being."

"And that means ..."

"Well, that I make mistakes."

"And that's okay because...."

"Well because human beings make mistakes."

"So what do you need me for? You have your answers! You know the solution."

"I know, but I still feel paralyzed by the fear."

"Are these two parts fighting inside of you? Are they at war within?"

"Not really. When I get paralyzed, I shut down and can't function."

"So the demand to be perfect is the superior game in your mind? It is the highest and is much more powerful than your realization that you are human."

"Yep."

"So do you have permission? . . . I want you to go inside and see. As you close your eyes and quiet yourself, say these words inside, 'I give myself permission to be human, to make mistakes.' And how does that settle inside you?" [Read the three dots . . . as a pause or silence.]

    "Okay. .. Well, kind of ... but not really."

"So are there any objections within you, within your mind or body to this permission?"

    "The objection is that I have to do it right."

"Oh, so you *have to*. *You have to*. Who says?"

    "Me." He said pointing to himself sheepishly.

"And so..."

    "It seems silly right now. Sometimes I feel like I have permission, but it doesn't last. It's temporary."

"Okay, so *you can do it*. And the problem is that it doesn't last. If I could hear that internal chatter, what would I hear, and how would I hear it? What does it sound like?"

    "Well, it is right here [pointing to the back of his head with both hands] in the two hemispheres."

"Well let's get some distance from those voices and objections, so if you imagine that voice moving from there down your neck and along your arms and down to your fingers, how is it when you listen to that objection when it is there?" [I gestured the movement and then was looking at my fingers and moving them and repeating the objection, 'You have to do it right.'] He did the same and took a couple minutes to imagine this.

---

* Jargon Alert *

Anchor: Any stimulus that you can use to trigger a response. An anchor can be any sensory stimulus (an image, sound, smell, touch). "Anchor" is used in NLP in the sense of a *trigger* for a Pavlovian stimulus.

"And what if we turn the voices into a whiny little thing, 'You have to do it right.' [I repeated using a nasal tone of voice.]"

    [Laughing] "That changes everything."

"Good, and what would you now need to believe so that you can fully accept yourself as a fallible human being who makes mistakes?"

    "I'm like everyone else — I am equal to everyone else. No one is better than anyone else; we are all the same."

"What decision do you need to make about that belief so that belief will lock in and be yours for the rest of your life?'

"I just need to decide. I will believe in the equality of all people."
"Good. And is that strong enough? Do you need anything else before we test this against the old triggers?"
"No, I need an anchor."
And with that he created an auditory anchor, the song— "We are the world."

Crucible Coaching
Would you like to be Neo—the new person in your Matrix world, *the one* who can master your Matrix so that you have it rather than it having you? As your Crucible Coach, I'll appear at the end of each chapter to work with you as your personal Morpheus. I'll be offering you red-pill—blue pill choices, I'll be pointing to doors that you can choose to walk through; and I'll be suggesting various challenges so that you can learn how to "free your mind." If so, then here's your first coaching assignment.

In your notebook, *My Transformational Life,* create a page with the title, "Awakenings." Now make your list. What have you been awakened to? What are some of your possibilities? What potentials clamor inside you urging you to begin to express it? What do you want to be unleashed from? What blocks and limitations to be freed from? What do you want to be unleashed to? What dreams call you into your future?

End Notes
1. The Matrix Movie came out after I had written *Frame Games* (1999) (now titled, *Winning the Inner Game*). That became such a useful metaphor, I created *The Matrix Model* in Neuro-Semantics in 2002.

2. To see the articles that I've written about *The Matrix Movie,* see the Neuro-Semantic website, www.neurosemantics.com. The titles are: Wake Up Neo the Matrix has you. Matrix Reloaded. Matrix Revolutions. Coaches of the Matrix.

Chapter 2

CHANGED FOR GOOD

Two Models of Change for
Unleashing Your Highest and Best

Have you ever tried to make a change, a significant life-enhancing change— and maybe you even achieved it for a little while, but then you slipped back? The change did not last. You didn't sustain the change because old patterns and old habits reassert themselves. Did that make you doubtful about change? About the reality of change? Did you begin to wonder: "How can a person change for good? How can a person change and keep the change?"

If so, that's great! *It's great because the Crucible is all about change.* It is about personal change, it is about group and cultural change. It is about how human stuff —the thoughts, ideas, beliefs, habits, response patterns, paradigms, understandings, operational styles, and so on—change in a transformative way. It is about how these things can metamorphosize into higher forms.

Today in a world where change is one of the most dependable and pervasive factors that we face, the Crucible enables you to take charge of the process of change so that you can keep up with it. This differs from the fact that most change happens *to* you whether you want it or not. You don't choose it; you don't guide and govern it. It's like being thrown off a speeding train, and then picking yourself up and chasing the train to hop back on! In the world of change, being able to adapt to it, to stay above the change, to anticipate it—these are the first important skills for coping effectively.

There's another set of change skills—those that enable you to intentionally embrace change. So in the Crucible, you are able to welcome change, guide it, work with it, and facilitate the kind and quality of change that *you* want. This addresses the opposite problem. In human life, we often wonder why we remain the same regarding some things and seem to not be able to change certain habits, ways of thinking, ways of feeling, or ways of being.

Here's a paradox. We are creatures of change, yet we sometimes feel stuck in not being able to make the changes that we desire and require. So what's the story about change? How does it happen? How can you take charge of the process and guide your own self-changes in ways that enhance your life and empower you individually? How can you more effectively operate as supportive change-agents to other individuals, groups, organizations, and cultures?

As a Neuro-Semantic process, *The Crucible Model* provides a way for you to take charge of the changes that you desire. It enables you to unlearn things that no longer serve you and to create a metamorphosis in those areas that will unleash new potentials so that you can be more fully alive, more human, and more authentic.

Kinds and Dimensions of Change
In answering these change questions, recognize first of all that there are numerous kinds of change and dimensions of change. When it comes to therapeutic changes, we are mostly speaking of *fixing* something that's not right, that's off-track, that's creating suffering, and that's distorted in some way. In the context of therapy, we want *a healing change* that remedies what's not right and that heals wounds—a *remedial change*.

Now the great majority of the literature about change relates to this kind of change—remedial change that brings healing to hurts, wounds, deficiencies, etc. And no wonder. This refers to a dimension of change where the *need* for change typically screams and hollers at you, especially as the

> *Remedial Change:*
> Fixing something that's broken or not right, creating a remedy for something sick or hurting.

current situation grows worse, becomes exasperated by the distortions, and puts you more and more out-of-alignment with reality.

There is also a really strange thing about remedial change—while you need it so much, and it would make so much of a difference in your life, you will typically fight it tooth and nail! Why? Because making this kind of change requires tremendous courage and ego-strength. So where there is any fear, low ego-strength, lack of internal resources (the very symptoms and indicators of the need for therapeutic change), human beings generally end up fighting and resisting the very changes they need. "That's crazy!" you say, and so it is. Well, from the outside. It's not so crazy from the inside perspective. From the inside where there are not enough resources to change —change seems and feels very dangerous. Consequently, people often think, feel, and say such things as, "Change is hard." "Change is painful." "People don't change easily." "I will never change."

In this area, those trained to deal with therapeutic change are prepared to expect *resistance* to the very changes that would make such a positive difference in their lives. They know to go easily and gently, to gain the trust and rapport of the person, to slowly invite and even seduce the person to catch a vision of all of the benefits that the change will bring.

> *Learning Change—*
> The change that naturally occurs as we learn; every learning changes us.

They know to expect the presence of the ego-defenses that will seek to fend off the change: denial, rationalization, projection, introjection, substitutions, excuses, etc. This is "the nature of the beast" when it comes to remedial change. That's one kind of change.

Another kind of change is *the change that we call learning*. This dimension of change is the ever-evolving and developing cognitive expansion and renewal of your map of reality. And this kind of change is most natural—it is part and parcel of how you are made. Born without "instincts" proper, we are a species that have to find and invent meanings which give us the content information for how to be human. Here you learn what a thing is, what it does, how it works, what it's good for, what significance it can have for you, etc.[1]

Change as a continually mapping and remapping your sense of reality ("learning"), typically involves experiencing the natural excitement and curiosity as learning becomes your way of life. Once you do this, then "school is never out." You become a life-long learner, as passionate in your thirties, sixties, and nineties for expanding your awareness as in the first years of life.

Another dimension of change concerns not only your cognitive growth and development, but the stages of your development as a person throughout the life-span. We call this *generative change* because it is about generating ever-new thoughts, emotions, and behaviors as you grow sexually, socially, interpersonally, in your performances, careers, etc.

People who embrace the ongoing development of *themselves* as *a person* through the stages of life experience generative change as the very adventure of life. And that is why they embrace change so passionately. People who enter into and embrace this area of change become *change embracers*. Rather than fearing change, resisting change, or thinking that it is difficult, change embracers look forward to the next step of their development and plan for changes. And when external changes come to them, they more quickly adjust to it with less upset or negative emotions. And because change represents the adventure and vitality of life, change excites them.

> *Generative Change:* Change that generates new responses, new ideas, new possibilities. The change of self-actualization that opens up new potentials.

Models of Change
In the book *Coaching Change* (2004), I identified several models for therapeutic change.[2] You know you are working with a therapeutic model because they are characterized by two unique factors: *resistance* and *relapse*. And given that therapy almost inevitably involves developing a stronger sense of self, self-value, and ego-strength, in remedial change the problem of the ego-defenses is a very real constraint to be addressed.

But what happens when a person gets to "okay," develops an empowering life script of "I'm okay; you're okay," and is ready to live that script by creating win/win relationships? What happens when a person is "up to average," has released the past, resolved past hurts, and no longer has an internal fight about one's gifts, strengths, weaknesses, and challenges? What then?

For the person who is now ready to take on life, to live life as an adventure of change, who is ready to become a change-embracer, and actualize his or her full potentials to become all that he or she can become—a different model of change is needed. Now we need a model that maps out how psychologically healthy people change and transform with grace, ease, and fun and that is the purpose of *The Axes of Change* Model.

The Axes of Change Model

The Axes of Change Model identifies four key mechanisms that facilitate self-actualizing change (growth or learning). The first loop is comprised of the motivation and the decision axes—these prepare a person for change. The second loop entails the creation and the integration axes—these make and solidify the change.

> **The Axis of Change**
> —
> **Loops of Change**
>
> *Preparation Loop*
> 1) Motivation
> 2) Decision
>
> *Implementation Loop*
> 3) Creation
> 4) Integration

Axis I: *Motivation for change* involves the polarities of attraction and aversion, pain and pleasure, toward and away from values. I say *polarities* because that's typically how we think and experience them even though each side works simultaneously within us. And if you embrace both sides of the polarities, you are then able to create a higher level synergy of both forces. When united together, you want *both* new pleasures and recognize the away-from aversions of not making the change.

Axis II: *Decision for change* involves the polarities of reflection and action, of weighing alternatives of the pros and cons and coming to mindful choice about an alternative that offers the best long-term enhancement of life. You create the synergy of cutting off some alternatives you are enabled to choose the best. You reflect long enough to make a smart decision and then make the commitment to go into a new direction and choice.

Axis III: The actual *creation of change* is also a two-fold process. It involves an inward and an outward focus. First you inwardly reference your game plan, your strategy, and your envisioned change that you give birth to through playing out your visionary dream of the new possibilities. Once you have created the basic structure of your inner game the time comes to take it outside to the real world. You make it your outer game in actual performance. The synergy you create here is between referencing things in the world of mind and then in the outside world. This explains why everything is created twice, first in the mind, then in behavior.

Axis IV: *Integration of change* plays off another set of polarities—that of supporting the fragile beginnings of change by looking for and honoring everything that fits or matches the inner game. In this, you treat the beginning of a new way of thinking, feeling, behaving, and performing as something fresh and young and delicate and so you treat it with care and gentleness. Then later, when there has been sufficient growth in the change, you can begin looking for whatever is not up to par to point out the differences, deficiencies, and inadequacies. Then you put them to the test and use that information to feed back into your inner creation.

With the four axes of change involving these processes, *the Axes of Change Model* identified eight change-agent roles whereby you can facilitate the process. These include Awakener and Challenger for motivation, Prober and Provoker for decision, Co-creator and Actualizer for creation, and Reinforcer and Tester for integration.

Change Agent Roles
1) Awakener
2) Challenger
3) Prober
4) Provoker
5) Co-Creator
6) Actualizer
7) Reinforcer
8) Tester

The Crucible as a Change Model
If *the Axes of Change* is one model in Neuro-Semantics for navigating the transformation process, *The Crucible of Self-Actualization* is a second one. What's the difference between these two models?

The Axes of Change Model is designed to answer the strategy question, "How do you know what to do, when, with whom, how, and why?" As such, it specifies four key change mechanisms and enables a change agent to engage in the *dance of change* with an informed awareness of the steps of the dance and how to follow a person's energy in facilitating generative transformation.

The change or metamorphosis that *The Crucible Model* facilitates answers a different question. It addresses the interference questions:
> "What do you do about old learnings that get in the way of new learnings?" "How do you *unlearn* what you have already learned and replace that which is now deeply ingrained within you?"

And rather than sorting out the mechanisms of change in a linear step-by-step fashion, the Crucible works in an organic and self-organizing way. The Crucible typically enables an intuitive and unconscious transformation of the mind-body-emotion system self-organizes and reforms in the sacred space.

To do this, we first facilitate the creation of a Crucible space. Using the metaphor of a crucible, as a holding place for transformation, we facilitate a guided imaginary for change. The metaphor itself arises from two sources, industry and artists. In both cases, a crucible is used to melt down iron ore and other elements which can then be poured into molds that give the metal new form and strength. The crucible is the holding space for all of this transformation of molten materials.

The imaginary here offers a powerful metaphor. Into a crucible you put unuseable things (metaphorically, iron ore) or things that are no longer useful and effective so that *the crucible operates as a holding space for transforming things.* As a metaphor of human transformation, a crucible is the space where you can hold your elemental components. Then, in that space you can face, witness, observe, search for positive meanings, and speak truth to yourself or another as a means for freeing yourself from old structures and for speaking a new world into existence.

The paradox of the crucible is that it itself does not melt down. Even though the crucible itself is made of fragile materials, it does not crack or shatter. Instead it holds the heat and the intensity of the experience and allows transformation to naturally occur.

The Crucible as a Change Model
When school psychologist Jim Walsh first experienced the Crucible Model and worked with it, he described the Crucible as a "change machine." "It's a machine to create change." I like that. Change occurs naturally and inevitably within the crucible. Holding a space where you can see reality in its intensity *and* feel supported as you face it *and* choose your best options, where you are not threatened at the level of self, all of this enables you to opt for your highest and best.

All of this also enables the Crucible to tap into and activate the principles of generative change within you—the principles of how you fully embrace change and use it for your self-actualization. What are these principles and the mechanisms of this kind of transformation?
- *Unconditional positive regard* distinguishes person and behavior, being and doing, person and experiences and thereby makes change safe. Now changes comes, not as a threat, but as a way to actualize your inner self and potentials. So the self-esteem of regarding yourself as having value and worth unconditionally makes it safe for you to change. By distinguishing your person from all of your expressions and experiences, you are able to eliminate personalizing. And if you are not personalizing the conditional things of life, then you will have no need to defend yourself. You are already okay, already a "somebody" that counts!
- *Witnessing* what *is* describes what you need to face. Now you can

address reality simply and neutrally. As this removes the fight, it eliminates your need for any ego defenses. This facilitates an openness to the world, to life, to reality. So the know-nothing attitude of pure observation (witnessing), non-judgment, and dealing with just the empirical facts increases your clarity. It enables you to see clearly without reacting, to align yourself with reality, and to adopt a reality-orientation in your approach to things. Now you can see yourself, others, and the world with innocent eyes!

- *Acceptance:* Acceptance is critical in the change process because you can't change what you don't accept. Acceptance comes immediately after witnessing and enables you to face and acknowledge whatever *is*. Acceptance, in the sense of acknowledgment, enables you to stop fighting, resisting, defending, and to release unrealistic expectations and demandingness.

- *Truth as reality:* Change, as the human adventure of growing and self-actualizing occurs through discovering and facing whatever is true, whatever is your truth at any given moment. This facilitates the development of clarity which leads you to focus on taking effective actions. Change occurs as you are ruthlessly honest in speaking the truth to yourself. By articulating what's real, authentic, and actual you are free to see, to understand, and to transform. Then you are free to be real. Being able to tell the truth establishes your credibility as it assumes that you are capable of coping with the world as it is without illusions, pretensions, and fantasy.

- *Truth as authenticity:* Because "the truth sets us free," learning to speak the truth compassionately and gently frees you to be real and authentic; it enables you to become a friend to reality, rather than an enemy to it. Also change is more often than not reorganization, rather than elimination. It's not so much a matter of making things go away as it is transforming them into new forms and expressions utilizing them in new ways.

- *Truth as confrontation:* You can never transcend what you do not confront. Typically, you change incrementally and developmentally as you learn to face, deal with, cope with, and eventually master the challenges and demands of life. You then transcend and include those experiences to learn from them and then move on.
- *Appreciation:* Valuing what's important, precious, and sacred transforms. As a meaning-maker, you live by meaning and

significance, so as you find and create value —you exercise your power of valuing, appreciating, and honoring what you previously feared, hated, misunderstood, etc. You then are able to transform even problems and distressful events into learnings that facilitate your self-actualization.

In appreciation you are able to see and recognize value, to "sacrilize" what is, create and attribute rich meanings. Finding and creating value enables you to honor many of the things that previously you would have discounted, feared, or even hated.

> You can't change what you don't own.

- *Ownership:* Embracing life as it is, and finding higher level *being*-values in it, changes you. Each and every "peak experience" touches you with the preciousness of life, of communicating, of relating and enables you to transcend yourself to serve others, to contribute, to make a difference in the world.

Taking ownership of your responses transforms so thoroughly because you step out of a victim state and into a creator's state. This also describes the pathway to empowerment since response-ability ultimately speaks about your response-*power*. To deny responsibility cuts you off from your basic human powers. Transformative change involves being accountable to others for your commitments.

- *Love, joy, ecstasy, peak experience, passion:* Why all of these words? Because they describe the effects of generative change. They give voice to some of the ways in which you will experience the change. And simultaneously these are also change factors in themselves. So, for example, falling in love with life describes a change factor. In fact, nothing is as transformative as the power of love. Love as *agape*-love, that is, benevolent good will toward others, toward life, and toward self provides an active, respectful, and healing power. This is the love that extend yourself for the growth, actualization, and development of others.

All of these words describes the love, the passion, the joy, the ecstasy that occurs when the generative change puts you in touch with that which ultimately inspires you. And because it puts spirit in you, it *inspirits* you, and creates a source of *inspiration* for you. And obviously in*spiration* changes people. To be inspired with an inspirational idea fills you with excitement, hope, purpose, meaning, direction. To be dispirited is to suffer existential discouragement. This is the transformation of "the peak experience" that Maslow identified at the heart of the zone of self-actualization.

Getting Ready to be Changed Forever

The Crucible is a place for radical and revolutionary change, it is also a place for gentle evolutionary change. Sometimes change occurs rapidly and suddenly like a quantum leap. And while it can be discontinuous, it can also occur as incremental change, the gentle evolutionary change that occurs as you grow and learn.

Crucible Coaching

Are you ready for a change? Are you ready to use the powerful change mechanisms described in this chapter to facilitate an unleashing of your potentials that will create a transformative change within you?

If so, then identify as specifically as possible what you want to change. What do you want to be unleashed from? And what do you want to be unleashed to? Get your blank notebook that you have titled, *My Transformational Life*. Now devote a page to the following theme: "I want to be unleashed from..." "I want to be unleashed to..." As you make an extensive list of experiences, thoughts, beliefs, emotional states, habits, behaviors, put a R for Remedial change and L for Learning change, and a G for Generative change.

End Notes

1. We are without "instinct" properly in the way that animals have instincts. See Maslow's classical work, *Motivation and Personality* (1954/ 1970) for a full explanation; also *Self-Actualization Psychology* (2008). Even if you don't consider yourself a "learner," learning is what you do all the time! Whenever you make sense of things and draw conclusions about life, you are learning.

2. See *Coaching Change, Meta-Coaching, Volume I* (2004) for a presentation of the Axes of Change Model.

Chapter 3

CRUCIBLES FOR AN ENCOUNTER WITH REALITY

"On the other hand, the kind of experience that you are having here [with these encounter groups] indicates that not only can people take honesty, but also that it may be very helpful, very therapeutic, it may move things faster. This is true even when the honesty hurts."
Abraham Maslow

Every *crucible is a paradox.* The paradox involves what it is and how we use it. In terms of use, we pour steaming hot metals, metals at the boiling point. And, yet in spite of the intense heat, the crucible maintains its own integrity as it holds the molten metals. Why do we do this? We melt the ore in the crucible so we can then pour that molten liquid into forms and molds to create new products. What is the paradox in this? The paradox is that most crucibles are made of fragile materials—clay graphite or silicon carbides. The paradox is that *the strength of a crucible lies in its fragile composition.*[1]

Crucibles used in art studios are so fragile that if you were to drop the crucible on a concrete floor, they would crack or shatter. So a crucible, fragile in itself, is yet strong enough to hold intense heat and energy. Pour molten bronze into a crucible and observe it swirling, burbling, hissing, and steaming. At that moment you are seeing and hearing potentiality in the making! These strong and resilient crucible vessels can profoundly change a raw substance and give birth to the creation of castings of various sorts.

This always elicits wonder, "What is the crucible made out of that it does not itself melt?" "How can it be so fragile and yet so strong?" And yet, as a metaphor for human transformation, there are other questions even more important that tease the mind.

Starting with the wonder of a crucible as part of the process of creating a work of art, we recognize that the essential job of a crucible is simple and singular—*to hold*, under extreme heat, *whatever is poured into it.* Using this as a metaphor, now wonder about the following:
- Is there a crucible for holding human experience?
- What could serve as a human crucible in unleashing potentials?
- Can we create a crucible for human transformation that would allow us to pour in our boiling hot thoughts and feelings, our passionate strengths, talents, visions, etc. so that we can form and create new expressions for ourselves?

If there is a human crucible, then what are the raw materials that we pour into it? Ah, yes, into such a crucible we will pour our emotions. And our thoughts. And our human drives and needs. And into it we will pour our needy emotions and wanting emotions. We will pour the emotions from our lower and higher needs, and also our unregulated emotions, our over-regulated emotions, our distorted emotions. Into it we can pour our impulses, struggles, virtues, fears, hopes, and a thousand other emotional responses.

Imagine pouring your emotions into a crucible and imagine seeing them become the swirling, burbling, hissing, and steaming stuff. Imagine your emotions as liquid energy from which you can find and create the shape of your unique passion and commitment. What is the crucible where you can allow such energy to bubble up and to burn off all dross making it more pure and uncontaminated? What will be the vessel for your hot emotions and raw passions? And what transformations can you then expect from this experience? These are the central questions for this model.

Building a Human Crucible

Before you can experience a transforming crucible for unleashing new potentials, you will first have to build it. How does that work? How do you build a crucible within yourself?

> "True freedom consists of accepting and loving the inevitable, the nature of reality."
> Abraham Maslow (1971, p. 119)

> *You build a crucible by the meanings you create about the experience of human transformation.*

Further, you build it in *the construct* of your mind.[2] The crucible for self-actualization will be built from your attitude of acceptance and appreciation for all your fallible responses. In fact, it is in knowing that your responses are but *expressions* of you, and not who you *are,* that enables you to accept, hold, and even *embrace your humanity in all of its fallible fullness.* Embracing this allows you to accept yourself without shame, embarrassment, apology, or guilt. You are a fallible human being. You are unfinished in your development, and you will always be. This is great, isn't it? And precisely because you are imperfect, you can be forever *becoming.* You can grow into ever increasing levels of authenticity.

Two attitudes or states that contribute to the creation of a human crucible are *acceptance* and *appreciation.* Fragile in themselves, these states enable you to embrace and hold yourself. By them, you able to hold all of your hot emotions, needs, passions, hopes, fears, etc. while you form and create new expressions in actualizing yourself. When applied to yourself, it is *self-acceptance* and *self-appreciation* that create the foundation for the Crucible. This gives you a way to even be a Crucible to yourself.

It is the just-observing attitude of acceptance that allows you to witness yourself without judgment. When you think about *acceptance* as a state of mind-and-emotion, it seems like such a small and insignificant state. It seems so fragile as a state. At first glance, it doesn't seem hardy enough to hold rage, despair, frustration, fear of self, self-contempt, etc.

Yet the power of acceptance is that it can enable you to *hold*, to just observe, to step back and see, really see, as you simply witness what *is.* Within this state you adopt a non-judgmental perspective. In acceptance, you don't condone, approve, want, desire, but neither do you resign or merely tolerate. Acceptance is more neutral and more positive. It acknowledges what *is* as well as welcomes what *is* for whatever it is, without needing to evaluate, judge, or reject.

If *self-acceptance* is what empowers you to create the foundation of a Crucible, then *acceptance* and *appreciation* of others is what enables you to become a Crucible for them. It is acceptance and appreciation of emotions-and-thoughts as just emotions and thoughts that creates the place where you can *hold* the energies that, in turn, unleash powerful potentials. Through *acceptance* you become a dependable Crucible for yourself and for others.

You can now hold emotions, no matter how hot, challenging, fragile or vulnerable the feelings.

Crucibles have the capacity to enable something to evolve in a new form from what has been old. Into the vessel of a crucible, elements are fused and transformed under intense heat and with highly focused energy. A crucible melts down old systems, refines out impurities, contains and refocuses energies, and sparks thresholds of change. Human crucibles are those experiences that often enable you to address and resolve some of the basic problems of existence. "Who am I? Where am I going? Who's going with me? What are my strengths, weaknesses, my potentials?" And, when used properly, you can use to forge solutions for how to live your life with meaning and vitality.

The Use of the Crucible

Besides bringing your hot thoughts and emotions into the Crucible, what else would you bring to and put into it? You could bring your hurts, wounds, sufferings, misfortunes, rejections, humiliations, abuse, violence, disappointments, and confusions. You could then let them enter to be changed and transformed in the Crucible. Would you like that?

> The most important thing about you is not your wounds!
>
> *You are more* than any and every emotional hell that you may have been through!

To do so is to recognize something critically important—namely, that the most important thing about you is not your wounds! Such experiences are just that—*experiences that you have been through.* They do not have to be your identity. Your experiences do not have to define you. Or more accurately, *you* do not have to identify yourself with the experiences you've been through or suffered.

You do not have to so identify with any particular experience and use it to define yourself. In fact, you can now bring your experience to the Crucible and *dis*-identify with that experience. That's because the truth is *you are more* than any and every emotional hell that you may have been through! You are no more a victim than you think you are, than you choose to believe you are. So, are you ready to give up any and all victim beliefs and emotions? If so, then the Crucible offers you an effective way to make that separation. After all, why suffer from the problem of defining yourself by your least resourceful moments and responses? Why build a monument to your worst moments?

When you use the Crucible you inevitably free up energy that's been devoted to holding down repressions and suppressions or other ego-defenses to memories, hurts, etc. you thought were dangerous to yourself. Over the years you have diverted your mental-and-emotional energy to keeping your inner hurts, memories, disappointments at bay. You defend your self against such.

For your self-actualization, you can also take your existential problems into the Crucible. These are the problems we all face regarding how to cope with our basic human drives. Maslow classified these under the emergent categories of the survival, safety, social, and self needs. *Emergent* here indicates that these needs are hierarchically structured. That is, each next higher need emerges as you adequately gratify the lower need. When you do that, the next level need arise. Human growth or development depends upon learning how to adequately and truly gratify the lower needs. These needs, driven by deficiency, fade away when gratified with "true gratifiers."

This keeps the drives healthy. There's nothing wrong with any of these drives. They reflect and indicate the actual requirements for life, for what we need to be healthy. And as *a true satisfier* truly gratifies the need, the drive remains healthy. Otherwise, the need can become unhealthy, even neurotic. What changes a basic healthy human drive into a neurotic need is a false satisfier. A satisfier is "false," when instead of gratifying the need so that it is satisfied and so vanishes and ceases to clamor, causes it to grow more demanding. A false satisfier first fails to gratify the need and second distorts the need so that it becomes ungratifiable. It's like drinking sand to quench thirst. The solution fails so thoroughly first in that it doesn't work and second in that it makes things worse.

How do you solve this distorting and neurotizing process? First, recognize it for what it is. Then identify a true gratifier. Construct in your mind a new understanding for how to effectively cope with the drive. This cleans up the mess and provides the inner healing that frees up the energy of that drive. In this, you can take unsatisfied drives and neurotic needs into the Crucible to have them restructured so that they serve your vitality.

Human drives and needs create the first levels of your values and are, by nature, organic. And to be healthy and integrated, they must come from the ground up. Is your need system strong, healthy, integrated, and whole? Are all of your lower needs as well as all of your higher needs healthy?

The Crucible is not only for hurts and traumas, you can even take your strengths into the Crucible. And why do that? The design is to mobilize your strengths, capabilities, resources, and powers. It is to activate your courage, openness, willingness to learn, and creativity. It is to summon up your powers to fight for your best.

Crucible Experience for Fear of Public Speaking
I held a Crucible space for Brenda when she wanted to release an old learning about public speaking. What the old learning was, she didn't know. All she knew was that even the idea of standing up and speaking causes her heart to pound, her lungs to begin breathing very fast, and her whole neurology to behave as if there was a great threat.

> "Okay, you can now just be with those feelings, unpleasant though they are, just be with them, and experience then so we can learn more about them, how you create them, and how to transform them."

As she then did that—following my instructions as she imagined public speaking, her body became tense as she tightened her muscles, her heart, and lungs worked harder and faster. As she did this I uttered words very quietly to facilitate the process. "That's right, and you feel that right now, and how intensely?"

She said it was at a level of 8 or 9. "Pretty intense, and you're just sitting here and there's no one here except me." I paused, then asked, "How old do you feel? Do you feel a different age than you actually are?" Surprised by the question and even more by her answer, she said, "Like two years old." I asked her to be with that, and go with that so that we could see where that would take her. "Now you're okay with this? Okay to allow me to guide you where you may not want to go?" She said she was.

> "Okay, so as you are with those sensations in your body and now let them take you whatever evoked them originally, just notice as you go there."

She was quiet for awhile, and her non-verbal responses was increasing in muscle tension as her heart raced.

> "I was in a hospital and being strapped to my bed, and my parents were not allowed to come into the room, they could peer through the window and watch me, and can only come to visit one time a week."

"Good, now step back from this so that you can see it without having to feel it. Just release the feeling and step back somewhere so you can see and understand." Brenda had bits of memory about that childhood experience of being in the hospital. I invited her to release it. "What is your truth about all of this that happened so long ago?" She said that it was "It happened a long time ago and is not relevant now."

> "So is there anything to save or keep from that?" [No] So are you ready to just let it go fully?" [Yes.] So as you do, just let your body release what it held on to..."

Maslow's Experience of a Truth Encounter
Maslow began to discover this facet of the Crucible toward the end of his life. He wrote about his new insights in *Farther Reaches* (1971).[3] The occasion was his visit to a rehab center in New York. He described it as *Synanon and Eupsychia* (Chapter 16). He there wrote about the intensity of the Crucible in the kind of "encounter" that people at the center experienced. In reflecting upon it, he wrote about his own experience in relating authentically and with brutal honesty to people.

> "I have spent a whole lifetime learning to be pretty careful with people, to be sort of delicate and gentle, and to treat them as if they were brittle china that would break easily."

It was there that Maslow saw and experienced what was called "an encounter group." Afterwards he spoke to the leaders of the Synonon group:

> "The assumption in your groups seems to be that people are very tough, and not brittle. They can take an awful lot. The best thing to do is to get right at them, and not sneak up on them or be delicate with them, or try to surround them from the rear."

He then commented that the experience of the encounter group at Synanon had called in question some of his basic beliefs:

> ". . . maybe [my] whole attitude is wrong. [Synanon] suggests that the whole idea of the fragile teacup which might crack or break, the idea that you mustn't say a loud word to anybody because it might traumatize him or hurt him, the idea that people cry easily or crack or commit suicide, or go crazy if you shout at them— that maybe these ideas are outdated." (p. 217)

Maslow described the encounter as getting —
> ". . . right smack into the middle of things right away. I've suggested that the name for this might be "no-crap therapy." It serves to clean out the defenses, the rationalizations, the veils, the evasions, and politeness of the world. In these groups people refuse

to accept the normal veils. They rip them aside and refuse to take any crap or excuses or evasions of any sort."

How about that? "No-Crap therapy!" From these reflections, Maslow then stepped back to reflect on what this meant about human nature:

"It raises a real question about the nature of the whole human species. How strong are people? How much can they take? The big question is how much honesty can people take? How is it good for them, how bad for them?"

As he wrote about in his reflections, Maslow then questioned T.S. Eliot's statement, "Mankind cannot bear very much reality." Once accepted, he then began to question this. His experience led him to contrast the idea that people cannot take it straight with the "encounters" at Synanon where they gave feedback to each other *straight,* pulling no punches.

"On the other hand, the kind of experience that you are having here indicates that not only can people take honesty, but also that it may be very helpful, very therapeutic, it may move things faster. This is true even when the honesty hurts." (p. 217)

"The things that people need as basic human beings are few in number. Do you think that this honesty, this bluntness that even sounds cruel at times, provides a basis for safety, affection, and respect. It hurts, it must hurt. The swords were out, and there was no gentleness about it. It was very straight, very direct, very blunt. Do you think that this works for you? Give out as much as they can take, dish it out, the faster the whole thing will move."

Then reflecting more about the role of responsibility in unleashing growth to "breed grown-up people," as well as the development of responsibility in the human personality, Maslow wrote:

"It looks as if one way to breed grown-up people is to give them responsibility, to assume that they can take it, and to let them struggle and sweat with it. Let them work it out themselves, rather than over-protecting them, indulging them, or doing things for them." (p. 220)

Finally, Maslow commented on the "normal" state of inter-personal interactions and communications:

"Nobody has ever been that blunt with me in my whole life. It is certainly a striking contrast to the conventional world, the world of university professors. It shook me up a little last night. In the world

I come from everyone is so polite because they are avoiding confrontation. There are a lot of prissy old maids around—I mean masculine 'old maids.'" (p. 224)

The fierce conversation in the Crucible invites you to be real in a whole new way than you've been before. You don't become authentic until you can honestly and truthfully face reality on its own terms. And you can't do that without the support of safety, value, compassion, and respect. When that's supplied, you have a Crucible. Then you can face the mirror which simply reflects back what is. You can then lay things on the line and get to the heart of the matter by *acknowledging the brute facts* without flinching. And this enables the unleashing of new possibilities.

Let there be Alchemy
The idea of a Crucible implies another metaphor—*alchemy.* In the middle ages of Europe, alchemy was a medieval speculative philosophy whose aim was to achieve the transmutation of the base metals into gold. Today we use the term *alchemy* for a metaphor of a power or process of transforming something common into something special. In the middle ages the hope was to transform lead into gold. These pre-scientists of that age were trying to figure out the secrets of chemistry to generate that kind of transformation.

Similarly, the gold of human personality, the gold of a person actualizing his or her highest values and best competencies is the alchemy that we seek via the Crucible. Here the creation is two-fold— de-construction and construction. First, the de-construction. Into the Crucible we invite lead and other raw materials of life so that it de-constructs it and creates new inner resources. Second, the re-construction begins when we give new form and shape to our energies.

Life often does this to us. Challenges in life often work as a crucible —bringing us into a self-encounter, bringing us to the end of an old way of being, and exposing us to truth, to reality, to love, to fear, to anger, to joy, to a wide range of emotions and dreams and visions ... and through it all boils down one way of life to bring into being a new way of being. In the lives of such persons of history as Moses, Jesus, Buddha, Joan of Arc, Martin Luther King, Nelson Mandela, Viktor Frankl, Christopher Reeves, and many others, an alchemy of personality occurred and history changed.

The crucibles in such cases tended to be hard, extremely challenging, and could have just as easy destroyed or wiped the person out as to have given birth to a transformative leader. *The Crucible Model* differs from this. It is not hard or rough at all. Like the release of nuclear energy that provides electricity for millions or within a nuclear submarine, the energy activated and released for new creation in the Crucible is under our control. We can form and reform it so that it works for our self-actualization.

Among the common lead of human experiences that we can now take into the Crucible and have transmuted into gold are old habits, old lifestyles, old thoughts, old beliefs, old emotions— creations of meaning that no longer serve you well. So if you are ready for a transformation, there's a Crucible ready for you.

Crucible Coaching
In your special notebook for your coaching experience, *My Transformational Life,* devote a page to "Ego Strength." Now answer the following questions:

>How strong is your ego-strength today? If ego-strength is the strength of your sense of self to face reality for what it is and to adapt and adjust and address that, how strong is your ego-strength now? Gauge from 0 to 10. (For more on ego-strength, see Building Up Ego-Strength, pages 43-44).

>What do you need as a resource that will strengthen this ability? Make a list of resources that will add strength, power, and energy to your sense of self.

>What do you believe? Do you believe that truth (what's real) is your friend or your enemy? Do you believe that you need to protect yourself from the truth or that the truth will set you free and enable your full development?

End Notes:
1. Fragile strength is just one paradox that arises from meta-stating. Others include glorious fallibility, playfully serious, curiously certain, or accessing your power bubble.

2. The "construct" here refers to your inner meaning-making capacity. See *Unleashed!* (2007). I devoted the first section of that book to an exploration of the human Construct.

3. Maslow, Abraham. (1953, 1971). *The Farther Reaches of Human Nature.* New York: Viking.

Chapter 4

WHY THE CRUCIBLE MODEL?

The Benefits and Elements of the Crucible

"The key concepts in the newer dynamic psychology are spontaneity, release, naturalness, self-choice, self-acceptance, impulse-awareness, gratification of basic needs."
Abraham Maslow (1970, p. 279)

What is the purpose of the Crucible? I hope that it is obvious to you by now. Given that I've been describing it as a place uniquely designed for transformation and metamorphosis—*the primary purpose of the Crucible is to facilitate generative change.* I also have spoken of it as enabling you to unleash hidden potentials so you can actualize your highest and best. So what else? What other purposes can the Crucible serve? There are several more that are central:

1) Unlearning old habits and unuseful constructs
2) Building up and developing your ego-strength
3) Dis-identifying yourself with limiting self-definitions
4) Finding and cultivating your true passions in life

Unlearning Unuseful Constructs
Learning is one thing. Then there is unlearning—an entirely different thing!

And sometimes it is *un*learning that we need most. *Learning* is actually our unique human "instinct." Given that we are born without innate knowledge about what to eat, how to cope, what to do, and even how to be human (without the kind of "instincts" that animals have), we have an opening in our mind—an area of not-knowing. It is an opening that allows you to learn your way of life—to discover and to create yourself and your unique expression of your lifestyle.

Now when you are born, you were an absolutely ferocious learner. Expose a child to any language, any culture, any context and he or she will learn it. And that child will learn it so thoroughly that it will set the frame for his or her thinking, emoting, speaking, and behaving for the rest of his or her life. It will become incorporated within that person's habits which will sometimes last a lifetime.

You are so effective as a learner that when you over-learn something, the learning will drop out of your conscious awareness and becomes what we call a "habit." When that happens, then what once required lots and lots of conscious attention and intention can now occur without thought. It occurs apart from your consciousness. In fact, now consciousness can mess it up. Now you perform complex learned programs automatically and without any awareness of what you are doing at all. From tying your shoes, riding a bike, typing on a keyboard, to using the grammar of your native language, and so on, you operate as if on automatic. This process offers a tremendous resource.

Yet it can also be a big problem. These old learnings, these habitual ways of operating, can now become problematic in terms of new learnings. Your habits can block new learnings. *So sometimes, you first have to unlearn what you have learned* in order to clear space and give yourself a chance to learn something new and different. If you don't, the new will be blocked and prevented from entering.

What is the significance of this? It is that your old habits frequently operate in ways that prevent you from changing. They operate as blocks to change. So first you have to clear the path by unlearning the habits that are no longer relevant for you. And what is a habit? A habit is a mind-to-muscle reaction as the answer to a problem or situation which now reduces your adaptability, resilience, and flexibility. The habit is an old learning that successfully solved one problem, but which now blocks you from moving to a new level of solution.

Now to unlearn past learnings, you usually have to reverse the process. You have to think again and think afresh. And that requires that you bring back into awareness what has been unconscious. To elicit creative thinking and become a bold thinker, you have to re-examine directly and freshly that which has become a habit.

This is where the Crucible comes in. As a place of change, it provides you an opportunity to do both—*to unlearn old responses and to learn new responses.* In fact, more often than not, you have to first unlearn so that you can then learn and creatively adapt a new response. What do you need to unlearn? What have you learned that now blocks your next level of development?

Unlearning Self-Pity
When I think about an example of an unlearning that occurred in the Crucible, I think about Philip. When I worked with him at a workshop, he told me that he needed to take "self-pity" into the Crucible.

> "Somehow early in life, when I was three or four, I think, I discovered that I could get people to do things my way if I went into self-pity and used it as a play. So I learned how to do that really well, and when I became a young adult, I took it to a whole new level of playing the victim. That was even how I would get women."

"So Philip, are you fully ready to take self-pity into the Crucible and let it melt down? Are you ready for it to be taken apart so that you don't use that as a way of coping in life to get your needs met?"

Philip said he was. I invited him to recall the special place that he had used when he constructed his Crucible and as he described the meadow in a upper New York area where there was a woods, a lake, and some small hills. He then went into the special state that he had created which enabled him to "be at his very best." I asked him to describe what he was seeing and hearing and feeling in that place, and then I asked him to notice how he had constructed and represented his sense of distinguishing self and behavior, pure witnessing, acceptance, truth, appreciation, and ownership. When that was completed, I facilitated the encounter.

"So Philip, with all of this in mind and fully feeling this very safe and protected spot, I want you to just witness things as you bring *self-pity* into this place and as you just witness it, see it, hear it, sense it, just accept that this was a set of responses that you had learned, and as you witness and accept it, what are you aware of?"

"I'm aware of how child-like and innocent the self-pity was when it started and how it grew to become more devious. I am aware that the self-pity was an accident."

"So Philip, is that your truth today? Is it that the self-pity started as an accident and that it was originally childlike and then over the years became devious? Is that true?"

"Yes. I didn't mean for it to become devious. I think that as I felt more and more insecure, it was a way of protecting myself."

"Ah, so is that your truth also? Insecurity drove the innocence of the self-pity and later it become devious. Is that your truth?"

"Yes. [Brushing away tears and laughing gently.] I guess I never realized before now that it just accidently grew, and it grew from insecurity, but that I let it lead me to become the insecure person I have become today."

"Hmmmm. So is that your truth? [Yes.] And given these truths, what can you appreciate about all of this?"

"Appreciate?"

"Yes. Okay, so now just move over to the big oak tree that over-shadows the lake in that meadow ... and in that place where you identified as where you put *appreciation*... What do you now appreciate about your self-pity?"

"Hmmmm. I have hated it for so long and had so much self-contempt about it ... hmmm ... this is hard... I can appreciate that it was at least an attempt at protecting myself."

"And what are you ready to *do* about this? What new responsibility are you ready to take on? Or perhaps, what are you willing to own that you have not owned before?"

[Pause] "I am ready to stop the self-pity ... and to be responsible for myself. ... Hmmmm. I am ready to stand up and assume full responsibility for myself and not excuse myself as I always have."

"Philip, is that your new truth today? That you will assume full responsibility for yourself and stop making excuses?"

"Yes, that's my truth today. I have had enough whining and acting like a little child when it comes to my responsibilities, and I'm ready to stop pitying myself for my inadequacies."

"And so what will you do, practically, from this day forward that will be

different?"
> "I will take responsibility for my finances, I will organize my bills and sit down and write checks for my bills when they arrive in the mail. I will also start an exercise program."

"That sounds like some new ways of being in the world. What do you appreciate about this?"
> "I appreciate discovering my powers, my four-powers of thinking, feeling, speaking, and acting and that my responsibilities are actually my response-powers. I really appreciate that."

"And..."
> "Well, it feels like a new lease on life. It feels exciting, and a bit scary, but what I want. Yes, definitely. What I want."

2) Building Ego-Strength

A second thing that you can use the Crucible for is to build up your ego-strength. What is ego-strength? How does it develop and how do we create it? How does the Crucible provide a place for building up ego-strength?

Ego-strength refers to the "strength" within your mind and heart about how you experience yourself so that you can simply face reality for what it is. It is the ability to face reality without caving in, falling apart, or reacting in either fight or flight. None of us have ego-strength when we are born. Ego-strength develops as you grow up, as you develop coping skills for handling your needs, learning to understand what things are, and how they work. The strength of your sense of self to accept things as they are and then exert the effort to deal with them develops and matures over the years until we have a sense of self-efficacy in ourselves to handle the challenges that life throws at us.

Obviously, witnessing, acceptance, truth-telling, appreciating, and taking responsibility are all ingredients of ego-strength. That's why the process of building a Crucible space within yourself and using it cannot but help to further your development of ego-strength. And yet what really enables ego-strength is the distinction between self and all of the factors and experiences of the self. When you make that distinction, you free yourself from feeling threatened by what happens to you or when you become aware of one of your fallible expressions.

Knowing that your worth, value, and lovability is unconditional, that it is a given, frees you to express yourself as you learn, make mistakes, and learn from them. None of this ever needs to call *you as a person* into question.

You are more than all of your fallible expressions. How you think, feel, speak, and act are just *expressions* of you, and not the ultimate "you." You are more also than what happens to you.

When I facilitated the process for John to go through the Crucible Model in New Zealand, he took into his Crucible his sense of inferiority. And each of the first dozen times that I asked him, "What are you now aware of?" he bristled inside. On the outside I could see him lean back, sometimes he jerked back as if startled. Later he told me that at first it was a shock to confront his inferiority. He said it felt like being hit with a bucket of cold ice water thrown on his bare skin. Each time I would remind him of his representations of unconditional positive self-regard, pure witnessing, and acceptance. Later he said that those works slowly linked the two together and enabled him to confront his inferiority.

3) Dis-Identifying with old Identities
A third benefit of the Crucible is that it can enable you to dis-identify with any and all (if necessary) previous identities that you have created. Sometimes, it is your old self-definitions and identifications that create the blocks within you that resist change and hold you back. You define yourself as being this or that kind of a person and eventually you embody and incorporate that identity so thoroughly that not only can you not imagine yourself differently, but any and every potential change to that identity is immediately rejected and resisted.

So if you have ever said, "Well, I'm not the kind of person who..." you have used an identity to resist a particular change or learning or experiment. In that case, the old identification stopped you from even considering operating in a new and different way. Taking that old definition of you into the Crucible will probably highlight the truth that you are more than your actions, experiences, group associations, skin color, religious beliefs, political affiliations, etc.

In this process you may discover new possible identities. After all, Who are you—really? Beyond your identifications, roles, and relationships, who are you in your authentic self? What are your truths?

That's when happened to Susan. She decided that her identity as a housewife was what she needed to unlearn. "Where did you put your Crucible, Susan? Where is the place that enables you to truly be at your best?"

"In the art studio that's in the upper room from the bookshop on fifth street. It's a beautiful place— full of windows and natural light, and full of all kinds of creative products and tools. And it looks out over a garden in the back."

"Great. Then if you close your eyes and go there now... just float ever so gently into that place of beauty and creativity and be there fully— seeing, hearing, feeling, and smelling that wondrous place." And after the guidance to that place, I invited her to refresh where and how she had encoded her Crucible space. Then we began. "Recognizing, as you know how to do, the distinction between your person and your expressions— bring the identity of being a housewife into this space ... [pause] and what are you first aware of?"

"I'm first aware of a tension in my body... in my neck and shoulders. And then I'm aware that this identity feels like body armor— like a iron suite, like the iron suits that knights wore in ancient Europe."

"And as you feel those kinesthetic sensations of that identity, what else are you aware of— other images, sounds, words, etc.?"

"I'm aware of my mother's voice, 'You'll never make a living as an artist; don't you know about starving artists? You need a good man to pay the bills; you should focus on just being a good housewife."

"Hmmmm. So now as you move, Susan, out to the balcony in the studio, your place of *acceptance,* and just feel the gentle feelings of acceptance so that you just acknowledge what is—what are you aware of as you just accept your mother's voice and words as *her* words and *her* voice?"

"Hmmm. It's strange. Those *are* her words.. her words and *her opinion* and, okay, I'll just accept that without needing to fully agree or argue with her. It's like I can hear her voice and that tone that always annoyed me, and leave it at that without it hooking me."

"Is that your truth?"

"Well, my truth is now that I don't have to sell myself short with a single identity. [pause] Yes, that's what I've done. I have sold my creative skills short all these years in order to be a housewife and to avoid taking the scary chance of making it on my own."

"So is that your truth— that you've sold yourself short and you didn't have to?"

"Yes."

"And so what are you now aware of?"

"That I can identify myself as an artist *and* as a wife, and housework

　　　　　　is just one thing I do."
"So are you more than a housewife?"
　　　　　"Yes!!"

"And with that truth, what responsibility are you ready to accept and own that will unleash your creative potentials?"
> "Well, I'm, already *doing* the art things, but I've never felt comfortable *being* an artist. My 'housewife' identity always blocked that. So now I will *be* the artist that I am."

"And what are you now able to appreciate in a new way?"
> "That I am really the one who gets to decide on how I identify myself." [Glowing]

"And what are you feeling right now?"
> "I'm feeling a radiance about myself that I have only felt about paintings and sketches! It's like I get to be the artist of my identity."

4) Discovering Yourself and Your Passions

Finally, a fourth benefit of the Crucible is that by entering it and exposing your habits, identities, needs, coping skills, thinking patterns, etc. to it, you can discover your passion (or passions) in life. That's what happened to Susan and it is what I have seen happen in hundreds of others. By allowing a new emergent self to arise— one which is unified, one-of-a-whole, new reverence for life engagement arises. You may find one or more passions in life to come to the surface.

Many people don't seem to know their passions. Dulled by expectations of others, the advice and suggestions of others, they have dulled their ability to hear their own inner voice. The voices of media, advertisements of what they are "suppose" to like and do have drowned out their own voice. No wonder they struggle to find an engaging passion in life. They can't hear their inner voice.

If that's the case with you, what do you need to unleash so that you can unleash your inner talents, gifts, and love? What interferes with hearing your own inner voice? What interferes from being the author of your own life?

The Elements of the Crucible

I mentioned earlier that I got the idea for the Crucible from extensively reading in the works of Maslow, Rogers, and other leaders of the first Human Potential Movement (HPM). Part of my searching was to discover and identify all of the ways that those of the first HPM found for unleashing potentials so people could self-actualize. And of all of the things that they found, one thing that they all seem to know and agree upon was that there had to be *an in-depth, authentic personal encounter.* They also knew of many of the healing and transformative qualities needed for that encounter.

In fact, the Encounter Group was the central "technique" of the Human Potential Movement. At Esalen and throughout the Growth Centers, T-groups and Encounter Groups—an encounter was used to help people encounter the issues that held them back from being fully authentic. But there was a problem with these groups. The encounter groups tended to be highly confrontative, in-your-face, aggressive, and very demanding. The result that most found them highly intimidating, even threatening and so defended themselves against the encounter. And that, of course, made them unsafe and likely to block the self-actualization.

The Crucible Model, as a new form of encounter, is designed to be a safe and respectful place that maintains the dignity of the person. True enough, the Encounter Group of the HPM did tap into several factors that serve self-actualization:
- Feedback for how you come across.
- Speaking the truth about your reality.
- Acceptance of self and others.
- Self-knowledge and understanding.
- And the universalizing human experiences.

But most of those Encounter Groups lacked other key components, most which had to do with creating a context where there was sufficient sense of safety and ego-strength for changing.

Learning from the first Human Potential Movement, I decided to design the factors and energies within the Crucible Model so they would be able to take turbulent emotions, desperate experiences, mind-numbing confusion and disruption, even dissipative forces and violence and forge something new out of them. What follows here is a brief overview of the elements of the Crucible that together are able to do this. Later there will be an entire chapter for each of these factors.

The Non-Directive Encounter
I began with the contributions of Carl Rogers (1951) who described the *kind of interpersonal space* for a crucial conversation. From his research he

described how to create safety and openness for what's deep inside for the person to emerge. Rogers' research led him to specify three items: empathetic understanding, unconditional positive regard, and authentic realness.

> *"My aim has been to provide a climate which contains as much of safety, of warmth, empathetic understanding, as I can genuinely find in myself to give."* (pp. 167-168)

This makes perfect sense, doesn't it? If we need a working space for potentialities to emerge and a space where we can work with the raw materials of our drives, needs, aversions, emotions, passions, wants, fears, dreams, etc., first and foremost we need a safe place. How do we create such a place?

Carl Rogers identified several critical success factors for awakening potentiality in his classic work, *Becoming a Person*.[2] What did he conclude was required and involved in becoming a person? Using his psychotherapeutic practice and case studies of people who were hurt and struggling, and even traumatized (his context was therapy) Rogers found that they need empathetic understanding, unconditional positive regard, and authenticity (genuineness, and congruency).

From this Rogers pioneered *client-centered therapy* based on the self-actualization premise that we are innately driven to grow, develop, and become. He believed that people can experience the process of *becoming*, that people have the necessary resources to do this, and that working with a client isn't about doing things *to* him or her, but facilitating a context, atmosphere, and relationship that allow the client to show the direction for his or her awakening and development. This is also one of the premises that NLP was later founded upon.

> "It is the client who knows what hurts, what directions to go, what problems are crucial, what experiences have been deeply buried. Unless I had a need to demonstrate my own cleverness and learning, I would do better to rely upon the client for the direction of movement in the process." (Rogers, 1961, p. 12)

Rogers, fully accepting the premises of self-actualization of Maslow, said that man is basically "positive" in nature, "is basically socialized, forward-moving, rational, and realistic" (p. 91). For Rogers, the variables that make for healing and transformation involve three essential factors and only three:
1) *Empathy:*
> Accurate empathy, empathetic understanding of a person which

accepts the person, understanding *with* a person and not just *about* him.

2) *Positive unconditional regard:*
A positive attitude of regard or esteem for the client as a person, all unconditional, that expresses a non-possessive love, care, or warmth for the person.

3) *Authenticity which includes genuineness and congruency:*
Being real, honest, and forthright about what one thinks, feels, and experiences in the relationship so that one is congruent in his or her communications and forthrightly honest in feedback.

Beyond Non-Directiveness

All of this works great for many people. Many people will naturally and inevitably self-actualize when these three elements are in place. But not everyone. Some people need more guidance. Some people need to know *how* to find themselves and their passions, and *how* to listen to their inner voice. Some need guidance in dealing with their interferences. Some people need to be guided in how to unleash their highest and best potentials.

Maslow discovered this toward the end of his life. Like Rogers, for years he expected that when people move up the hierarchy of needs and reach the place of being able to effectively gratify their needs with true gratifiers, they would then naturally and inevitably evolve to become self-actualizing people. They would then live at the level of the *being*-needs. But then he found himself teaching in a wealthy private University populated by a lot of rich kids— young people who had all of their lower needs fully gratified, and then some. And yet they did not move on to the characteristics, values, or lifestyle of self-actualizing people. Why not? What prevented them from self-actualizing?

That's when Maslow discovered that, with some people, the non-directive approach doesn't work. The process of choice for how to proceed isn't to be left to their own devices. They need guidance. So when I discovered that, I began looking for some additional elements that would have to be in the personal encounter of the Crucible. That's when I found, in Maslow's work, some additional ingredients that would complete the encounter —truth, appreciation, and responsibility.

In *Toward a Psychology of Being,* I discovered that Maslow wrote the following about self-actualizers:

"They could let themselves be flooded by emotions. ... In trying to figure out why all this was so, it seemed to me that much of it could

> be traced back to the relative *absence of fear* in my subjects. . . . They seemed to be *less afraid* of what other people would say or demand or laugh at. They had *less need* of other people, and therefore, depending on them less, could be less afraid of them, and less hostile against them. Perhaps more important, however, was their lack of fear of their own insides, of their own impulses, emotions, thoughts. They were more self-accepting than the average." (*Toward a Psychology of Being,* p. 140, *italics added*)

If the encounter involves strong emotions and a person is afraid of his or her emotions, then that person will need support and guidance in the experience of being "flooded by emotions." That person will need support and guidance in getting over a fear of self (which is a negative meta-state). The dynamic that often creates limitations that leashes us and that prevents self-actualization is *fear* of self and *protection* against self.

> "By protecting himself against the hell within himself, he also cuts himself off from the heaven within. ... As a consequence, more of themselves is available for use, for enjoyment, and for creative purposes. They waste less of their time and energy protecting themselves against themselves." (p. 141)

This again identifies the importance of having some direct guidance for getting beyond one's ego defenses.

> "The principal reason the self-actualizing person sees reality more clearly is that they see it through an unclouded lens [clean cognizing and meaning-making]. They place no unrealistic, neurotic demands on reality [cognitive distortions]. It is not only that self-actualizing persons seeing the world as it really is, *they also accept it as it really is.* The result is that they are more comfortable with what they see and less fearful of what they do not see."

When it comes to the whole realm of thinking distortions, mental habits of thought that create misery, these habits are often so unconscious that we're completely unaware of them. They make up our blind spot. And as blind spots, they undermine our ability to confront ourselves with truth.

Another quotation from Maslow (as quoted by Richard Lowry) highlights the importance of embracing uncertainty and ambiguity:

> "Our healthy subjects are uniformly unthreatened and unfrightened by the unknown, being therein quite different from average men. They accept it, are comfortable with it, and, often, are even *more* attracted by it than by the known. They not only tolerate the

ambiguous and unstructured; they like it." (Lowry, Richard, 1973, p. 41)

Again, many people, if not most, will need guidance and direction in this. They dislike ambiguity, confusion, chaos, etc. and so immediately seek to escape. They do not know how to enter and go through them.

"Looking within oneself for many of the answers implies taking responsibility. That is in itself a great step toward actualization. . . . In psychotherapy, one can see it, can feel it, can know the moment of responsibility. . . . This is one of the great steps. *Each time one takes responsibility, this is an actualizing of the self.*" (1971, p. 45, *italics added*)

Finally Fritz Perls, another pioneer in the first HPM, focused on the importance of being present in the now—in the moment— as one of the central themes of Gestalt therapy.

"Without awareness, there is no cognition of choice. Awareness, contact, and being present are merely different aspect of one and the same process—self-realization." (1971, p. 66)

The Crucible Model
While there are seven elements to the Crucible as a model, it also has three stages: the preparation, the furnace, and the transformation. Three of the elements come together to create *the preparation*—the safety (unconditional positive regard, witnessing, acceptance). Three additional elements work together to create *the furnace* where the heat and intensity of the Crucible occur (truth, appreciation, responsibility). And then one element results that indicate *the transformation* of the Crucible (love, joy, ecstasy, peak experiences).

1) The Preparation Stage
You have to prepare yourself to enter the Crucible. Unprepared with the proper ingredients, and the Crucible encounter will only evoke a sense of threat and danger. That will undermine one's awareness and create a level of blindness. The quality of your awareness creates the quality of what you see and experience. Fear prevents entry to the Crucible. Typically, you are either not safe enough to enter or strong enough. Your ego defenses and ego escape mechanisms prevent you. Given this, to enter you need three qualities—witnessing to observe, acceptance to acknowledge what is, and unconditional value for individuals so that what is seen and observed do not take away from one's personal value.

2) The Furnace Stage of Encounter
The heat of the furnace is truth. Survival personalities and identities need to go into the crucible so you release and give up these false selves. Untamed emotions can include what you call your "dark side," your sense of loss of self, your fear of non-being, or of being overwhelmed, or possessed. This may involve a place of silence, presence, patience, of being with something, being in the moment. It also includes valuing—seeing value, clinging and enhancing meanings, sacrilizing, and releasing dis-values.

When you change the quality of your awareness and attention; you change your perceptions of yourself and others. When you truly come home to yourself, you transform. If you reject a particular feeling, "I don't want to feel this." You feel threatened. Rejection is a form of violence against yourself. Judge yourself or your feelings and that blaming perpetuates the situation.

3) The after-glow
From the furnace comes a new passion, the passion of falling in love with life again, falling in love with certain activities, with expressing your true self, your creativity. The nobility of the human spirit — in acts of kindness, courage, self-sacrifice, and compassion.

The Place where you are at Your Best
How do you imagine a Crucible? If you google "crucible" you will see that it is a container— some small, some large, some gigantic. Some are like a small bowl you can hold in your hands, others are like a vat, and yet others are the size of a building! To this point I have also used some other words and images— furnace, fire, oven. Perhaps you entertain images of a sweat lodge, a witches kettle (!), or a desert wilderness. Of course, the problem with these images is that none of them feel very safe!

So to counter-balance all of this, let's put our crucible space in a place that brings out your best. To find your place, scan all of the places in your mind— real or imagined— that *when you are there, you are at your very best.* In what geographic place do you truly come alive? Where do you love going that rejuvenates your spirit, that makes you feel, "It's good to be alive!"? Where is the place that enables you to feel free to turn loose and relax in who you are and what you have to offer? That's the place that we will transform and commission as your Crucible space.

Crucible Coaching
It's coaching time again. So get out your notebook, *My Transformational Life*. Now at the top of a new page, put the title, "Unlearnings: Things to Unlearn."

> What do you think you need to *unlearn* in order to be free to learn afresh and continue your development to unleash your very best self? What habits of mind, emotion, or relationship now block your full development? After you have written your list, ask two or three people who know you well what they would suggest.
>
> What identities have you created, developed, or adopted from others that are now ineffective and no longer serve you? Do you know how to dis-identify from those old identities? Are you ready to do so?
>
> Next, create another page on "Unlearning Skills." What unlearning skills do you have now? What unlearning skills do you need to learn? Of the following unlearning skills and patterns, which do you need to learn or experience? Do you need to learn how to— ?
> - Suspend meaning
> - Release frames
> - The Drop-Down Through pattern to release embodied frames[1]
> - Deframe

End Notes:
1. You can find the Drop-Down Through Pattern on the Neuro-Semantics website in one of the articles on stuttering, www.neurosemantics.com.

7 Key Elements of the Crucible

From Maslow, Rogers, etc.   *The Crucible of Transformation*

1) Unconditional positive regard   —   Distinguish person/ behavior

2) Accurate empathy   —   Witnessing, awareness without judgment

3) Acceptance   —   Acknowledge and welcome what *is*, open

4) Authenticity, personal congruence —   Speaking the truth, being real, facing what's real

5) Responsibility   —   Ability and willingness to act, to respond, to own responses

6) Appreciation to see and add value, to sacrilize   —   Appreciation of the values, benefit, and positive intentions

7) Peak experiences of pure joy and love   —   Love (benevolent good will to give of oneself), passion, humor, sense of transcendence

Chapter 5

TRANSFORMING EMOTIONS

IN THE CRUCIBLE

Self-Actualization and Your Emotions

*"So this too must be studied, this fear of human goodness and greatness,
this lack of knowledge of how to be good and strong,
this inability to turn one's anger into productive activities,
this fear of maturity and the godlikeness that comes with maturity,
this fear of feeling virtuous, self-loving, respect-worthy.
Especially we must learn how to transcend our foolish tendency
to let our compassion for the weak generate hatred for the strong."*
Abraham Maslow (1968, p. iv)

A Crucible for Hot Energies[1]

There's a funny and paradoxical thing about *emotions*—handle them right and they powerfully facilitate the *unleashing* process, but mishandle them and you will not only miss out on the unleashing, your emotions will get a iron-grip lock on you. And if that happens, they will lock you into a prison of negativity and defensiveness. They will shackle you to your fears, worries, and guilts. They will operate like devastating fire-breathing dragons to you.

Your needs, impulses, and emotions are the raw materials out of which you create and transform the development of your personality. There is an unleashing power in your emotions that facilitates your self-actualization

growth.
- The joyful gratification in satisfying your basic needs.
- The excitement of the transcendent meta-needs that takes you to a whole new level of experience.
- The fascination of exploring your strengths and weaknesses.
- The focus and engagement in experiencing the flow state.
- Welcoming and using a weakness for self-discovery.
- Feeling bad, even guilty, and using it to discover a wrong action to change.
- Feeling the release through forgiving an old hurt.
- Feeling centered and grounded in a solid sense of self, self-confidence in what you can *do*, self-esteem in what you *are*.
- The enjoyment of fully expressing your potentials.
- The awe of becoming more fully yourself.

In these ways, and many more, your emotions support, enhance, and empower you in unleashing more and more of your potentials. Yet you also have to face the backside of your emotions—emotions can just as equally undermine and diminish your potentials. You can suffer an imprisoning effect by the effect of living in your negative emotions, in stress, frustration, confusion, shame, fear, anger, etc. All of this underscores the importance of handling your emotions intelligently.

To jump to warp speed with your higher needs as you unleash your potentials, you need energy. And because much of that energy comes from the energy of your emotions as emotional states, *unleashing* demands tapping into the power of your states.
- How can you most effectively manage your emotions?
- What emotions facilitate the unleashing of potentials?
- Which emotions undermine self-actualization and lock up your potentials?
- How can you best handle those emotions to use them in the unleashing process?

This is not a new realization. We have long know that emotions play a key role in unleashing as do cognitions. More recently, we have become aware, through the work of John Mayer and Peter Salovey (two psychologists who coined the term), Daniel Goleman, and others, *the extent to which emotional intelligence plays a critical role* in our lives, relationships, and success. What isn't so clear yet is *how* to most effectively understand your emotions, the roles that they play in unleashing your vitality, and how to mindfully manage them.

Embracing and Holding the Emotional Energy of Emotions
- What role do emotions play in the releasing of your potentials for self-actualization?
- How should you think about your emotions in the self-actualization process?
- What meanings do you need to develop about emotions to support the unleashing of potentials?

Your emotions primarily are all about a somatic signaling of your energy system. You feel emotions in your body as *action tendencies* that get you to move (*motion*) out (*ex-*) in response to whatever is occurring and triggering your emotions. The content value of the emotion is what tells you that there's a positive or negative *difference* between what you've mapped about reality and what you're experiencing.

Did you get all of that? I know that it is a really loaded statement that describes what emotions are and where they come from. So here it is again, a little slower and in some different words.

An emotion is *the difference* in your body (soma) between what you have mentally, in your mind, mapped out about life, self, others, and reality (your meanings and semantics about any given thing) and what you actually experience, given your skills and the particular context.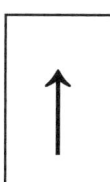
    If that difference is positive—you feel positive and sense that your mapping is accurate, or at least useful. The positive feelings represent a validation of your maps which creates the "positive" correlation.
    If that difference is negative—you feel a negative feeling and you sense that your mapping is dis-validated. The map is invalidated as not right, that is, it does not work for what it's designed to do.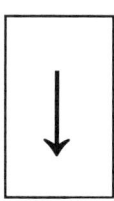

Overall what this means is that any and every emotion is always right. *It is right given the map from which it comes.* But it is not always right to the territory. In fact, it can be very, very wrong and misleading.

A good image for this is a balancing scale.
    On one side you have your *semantics*—all of the meanings you have

constructed as your maps, understandings, expectations, beliefs, values, decisions, imaginations, memories, etc. These meanings map your perceptions.

On the other side you have your *experiences*—your performance, actions, and behaviors, skills, conversations, interactions with others and with situations (according to your map). One side is the map, the other side is the territory (actually, your experience of the territory).

One side is the map of expectations, the other side is your experience in the territory using your skills. When your mapping is equally matched with your experience, your external world and internal worlds balance nicely. When this happens, there's little difference. And with little difference, there is little or no motion (or emotion). Things feel as they should. So there's no urge within to "move out." There's no place to move out to or from. Because you are experiencing things as you have mapped them, all is well with your world.

When your mapping is validated and confirmed, there's difference, positive difference, and so you feel the "positive" emotions. Here the scale of the world out there goes up, giving you more than you mapped. You feel delight, joy, love, wonder, surprise, curiosity, celebration, fun, trust, excitement, etc., the joy is that your maps work to navigate where you want to go. It's time to put "the pedal to the metal" and "floor it" as you speed down the highway of life.

When your mapping is dis-validated and disconfirmed by experiences that fail to confirm your ideas and by experiences that prove you wrong in your thinking, your maps are threatened. So you feel under assault. You feel angry, afraid, disappointed, disillusioned, sad, guilty, wrong, etc. Here the scale of the world tips downward. The world isn't giving you what you mapped. Something is wrong. It's time to check the engine, the gas, the oil, to stop, look, and listen for what's wrong that creates the incongruency between mind and experience.

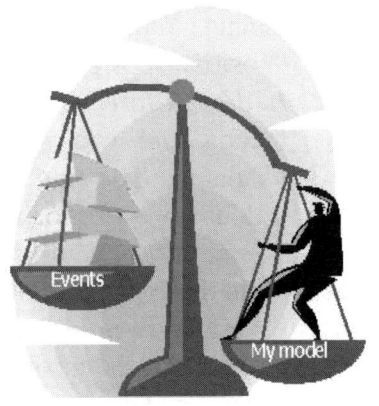

What occurs in your body (soma) are the

psychosomatic urges and *motions* that *move you to act*—to do something about what you're feeling. In the positive emotions, you feel moved to continue on your trajectory, and to do more of the same. In the negative emotions, the energy moves you to "stop, look, and listen" and to make a change, to stop whatever you are doing, and to find out what's wrong with the map or with your skills in navigating the territory. Like the nerves in your body, some are excitatory and some are inhibitory.

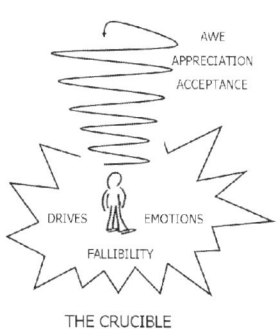

In both instances, positive and negative, your emotions are powerful forces for unleashing energy, mobilizing new resources, and energizing you as you pursue your goals and objectives. As such, your emotions need to be fully embraced. And this introduces a second great shock:

> *Emotional intelligence begins when you can now accept all of your emotions.*

And accepting enables you to use all of them as sources of information —information about how well your thinking (maps) enable your navigational experiences in the world. At the same time, *they are as just emotions.* Negative emotions move you to change something—either your mapping of things, or the way you're attempting to move forward.

William James (*Psychology: A Briefer Course*) recognized the power of emotions and asserted that we need to detect emotions as they arise, then tap into them to use them for developing our response patterns:

> "When a resolve or a fine glow of feeling is allowed to evaporate without bearing practical fruit, it is worse than a chance lost; it works so positively to hinder the discharge of future resolutions and emotions. Never should we suffer ourselves to have an emotion . . . without expressing it afterward in some active way. Let the expression be the least thing in the world . . . "[5]

What if you don't feel anything? What if most of your feelings are negative? Then you probably need to take your foot off the brake. What if you are over-emotional? What if you are highly sensitive to emotions? Then it will probably be good to take a fresh look at your mapping—your expectations, thinking patterns, and meanings.

All of this leads to more exploration questions for unleashing your potentials:
• How well adjusted are you to all of your emotions, positive and negative?
• How well do you accept, appreciate, and embrace your emotions as the impulse engine of your potentials?
• Are there any emotions that you do not accept and embrace, but fight and resist?
• What are the most empowering belief and value frames that will enable you to more fully welcome your emotions as just emotions?
• In terms of emotional intelligence, how high would you gauge your E.Q.? (E.Q. entails emotional awareness, acceptance, monitoring, regulations, elicitation, and use for connecting or relationships.)

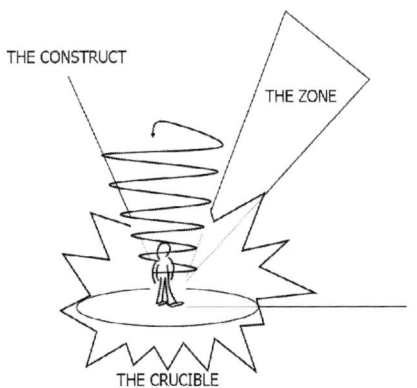

Crucible Creation — the Holding Power

If the energy and power to *unleash* hidden potentials arise from your emotions, then how do self-acceptance, self-appreciation, and non-judgmental awareness become the Crucible that holds this energy? How do acceptance, appreciation, and witnessing become the place where you can simply let your emotions be without judgment or fear? How do acceptance and appreciation give you a place for molding and shaping your emotions and emotional responses?

These questions take us to *the Construct*—to the *meanings* that we construct about emotions.
• What do you believe about your emotions?
• What do you believe about the expression of your emotions, about your anger, about your fears, etc.?
• When you think of "getting emotional," what thoughts and feelings and/or memories or imaginations come to mind?
• What have you decided about even exploring your emotions?
• What emotions are prohibited and tabooed for you?
• What do you believe about accepting your emotions?
• What do you believe about acceptance?

As you answer these questions, *your answers make up your Crucible.* Your answer describes your current Crucible. That's right. If you don't allow crying and tears because you believe "sadness is weak," or "boys shouldn't cry," or "be strong, crying allows others to take advantage of you," then you have a Crucible made of ideas that will weaken and diminish you— ideas that will not be able to hold the intensity of sadness. You will avoid sadness and if you give in to feeling sad, you will fall apart.

For you, as for all of us, your *Crucible* arises from the meanings that you create about emotions and particularly about your acceptance or rejection of your emotions. Your matrix of meaning frames gives you the power to be with your emotions and those of others, or that limits and prevents you from just witnessing them. If you dislike your emotions, if you shame yourself for feeling in any certain way, you create a Crucible that will easily melt, crumble, and collapse.

Crucible or Defense Palace
To understand the Crucible, contrast it with your defense mechanisms. After all, what do you do when you feel threatened and go into states of defense or escape? Do you not rationalize, explain, deny, project, introject, fantasize, blame, etc.? You step into a mental-and-emotional space inside yourself where you defend and protect yourself from reality, from the facts of your nature and experience. It's your fortress of escape and defense. You wall yourself away from your emotions and drives by pretending, wishing, and running away. Inside that castle of denial and defensive, you also freeze the things that frighten and threaten you. Rather than face and deal with the source of threat, you lock up your emotions, drives, fallibility, and so your humanness. You put these things under lock and key. But, of course, they don't go away. They grow in your apprehension and anxiety. It is in this way that you create "dragons" within.

The Crucible is the very opposite. Here is a living, breathing boiling cauldron of thoughts-and-feelings that acknowledge, welcome, accept, allow, and permit whatever *is* to just be what it *is* and to do so without judgment or censor. *The Crucible is a place for truth, for truth-telling, for being ruthlessly honest about whatever **is**.*

Do you fear and resent your masculinity or femininity? Do you fear and reject your anger or fear, your worries and jealousies, your negativity and hate? In the Crucible you acknowledge these human feelings and drives as *just human stuff.* In fact, rather than judge and hate and censor, you see that these experiences are actually good, even desirable. Anger has its place; so does lust, even hate. Actually, these emotional powers are wonderful, even beautiful. In the Crucible you learn to delight yourself with these human energies and awarenesses. You learn to stand in awe of them. You do so by releasing your demands that they be otherwise, that things be "perfect" in a way that's not humanly possible.

The Transformational Process

One of the things that primarily troubles most people are their negative emotions. Yet while they give us the most grief, you can also be deeply troubled by your positive emotions. Of course, to be emotionally intelligent, you will want a strong and powerful relationship to both your positive and negative emotions. The paradox of unleashing potential is that you best release your negative emotions by fully accepting and embracing them. By welcoming them, they lose their power to shock and overwhelm you. What is the secret here? It is to never turn a negative emotion against yourself. That's what causes the trouble and creates "dragon states."[3]

In Neuro-Semantics we describe this principle in this way.

> *When you bring negative emotional energies* (negative thinking and feeling) *against yourself* (or against any conceptual facet of yourself) *you put yourself at odds with yourself.* Doing this turns your psychological energies *against* yourself in unuseful, non-productive, and typically toxic ways. It creates the unresourceful states or "dragon states" of self-attack and self-abuse.

To frame or meta-state yourself with acceptance, appreciation, honesty, and non-judgment, use the following pattern. As always, it is best to have someone coach you through it by asking the questions and supporting you in discovering and creating your Crucible.

The Meta-Stating Pattern

1) Identify an emotional state with which you have difficulty handling, controlling, or managing.

> Your menu list may involve negative emotions such as anger, fear, disgust, regret, bitterness, etc., it could involve even positive experiences such as feeling sexual, being sensitive, feeling tenderness, vulnerability, etc.
> What negative emotional state of thought-and-emotion do you not like, can't stand, hate, wish you didn't experience?
> What negative states do you feel as *taboo*?
> What emotions or thoughts are prohibited within you?

2) Check and give yourself permission.

As you quiet yourself, take a moment, perhaps to close your eyes and say within your mind, "I give myself permission to feel X."
Notice any internal responses that might arise as you say this.
How well does that settle inside?
What objections, if any, arise to this?
What resources would you need to access in order to more fully accept this?
What reframe of meaning would you like to add to this experience?
Have you given yourself permission congruently with a strong and resourceful voice so that it reframes the objections?
How does that settle inside?

> "I give myself permission to feel anger because it allows me to recognize things that violate my values and to take appropriate action early."
>
> "I give myself permission to feel the tender emotions because it makes me more fully human."

3) Set a meta-state or frame over the negative emotion or experience using acceptance, appreciation, and other powerful resources.

Access each and fully apply acceptance, appreciation, and perhaps also calmness, thoughtfulness, fallibility, playfulness, and whatever other resource you need. Because you want to access *the mind-body feeling state* of these, use small simple referents. *Acceptance* is not resignation or condoning, it is welcoming and acknowledging what *is*.
What do you now easily accept?
What do you accept now that you may have once rejected and hated, but now just accept? Do you accept taking out the garbage, driving in rush hour traffic, a rainy day, etc.?

4) Quality control the resource frames.

Imagine fully and completely moving into your tomorrows with this frame of acceptance and appreciation regarding your negative emotion . . . are you fully aligned with this? Does any part of you object to letting this operate as your orientation style? If so, recycle back to adding in the sufficient resources that you need.

5) Put into your future and install with a meta Yes.

Would you like this to be how you move through the world?
Are you willing to make this your orientation?
Would this empower you as a person?

Would it enhance your life?

Releasing Your Brakes
There's another metaphor that I like regarding emotions. I like to compare the positive and negative emotions to a car's pedals for acceleration and braking.

The positive emotions accelerate—they give you the energy to accelerate, to "go for it." The positive emotions say:
> "What you are doing is working, they fit your mapping about reality and things, so do more of the same."

The negative emotions brake— they give you the braking energy to inhibit and restrain what you are doing. The negative emotions say:
> "What you are doing is not working, is violating the way you have mapped things. Stop now! Look, listen to what's going on and do something to make the necessary corrections."

These messages may be accurate or not, appropriate or not, timely or not. That depends on the difference between map and territory content that the emotions are registering. Given that your emotions have a signal value according to the difference between your map of the world and your experience of that same world, sometimes they offer wonderful insights, sometimes they are the epitome of stupidity. That's because as you can misunderstand and mis-believe, you can mis-feel.

How do your emotions contribute to the unleashing of potentials process? The positive emotions, that you feel when fulfilling your basic needs, create your basic propulsion power to move forward. They enable you to step up to the higher needs. The positive emotions coming from your self-actualization needs creates within you a warp-drive engine.

Your negative emotions provide an important and great service when they accurately indicate problems. A potential problem, however, is that if you *live in* the negative emotions, they will become habitual. They then become your habitualized frame of mind, and you will then live with the brakes on(!). You will be trying to get on down the highway of life riding your brakes. This describes what so many people experience in life and explains why they are not actualizing their full potential. They are driving with the brakes on. This clearly identifies one thing they need to do. To unleash their potentials, they need to *release the brakes!*

Put the positive and the negative emotions together and you can create a *propulsion system* within your personality to jet-propel you into the warp drive of your self-actualization. Then you will have both the *push* and the *pull* energy working together, moving you *away from* aversions and pains and *toward* attractions and pleasures.[4]

Using Your Emotions to Unleash Your Potentials

- Your emotions are secondary, not primary. When you believe and treat them as primary, you use the power of your Construct to semantically load your emotions so that they *have* you rather than you *having* them. This creates unnecessary limitations and leashes your potentials.

- Your emotions are *action tendencies in your body* that make you want to move, to do something, to get away, to attack, to do something so that you alter your state. *E(x)motions,* as action tendencies, are designed to give up power and energy "to move out" from where you are and take care of challenges.

- The moving-out feeling of an emotion is just a somatic urge in the body that comes from the *difference* between how you have mapped something in your mind and what you are experiencing in the outside world. As the difference between your map and the territory, it is *real* inside your body, even though it is not real in any ultimate sense.

- As you create a Crucible of acceptance, you can now use your emotions as a true propulsion system so that you experience a turbo charged energy moving you forward.

Making it Personal

I remember the first time I simply acknowledged an emotion that had been tabooed in my life and that seemed completely outside of what was acceptable. At twenty-three I was faced with some challenges at work regarding my competency. As a result, I was fired. The sense of loss that came with that particular firing was immense because I loaded it with so many meanings. So, experiencing and feeling some very significant losses, I naturally felt sadness and grief, perfectly normal reactions and emotions.

Except, inside the matrix of my mind at that time, they were not normal. They were not acceptable at all! In fact, they violated the very foundations of my sense of self, of my masculinity, and ability to cope in the world.

After all, I had well integrated some pretty toxic ideas in growing up. "Boys shouldn't cry" my dad taught me. As a World War II Sergeant, he had drilled that idea into me, "It's a cold world out there; have a stiff upper lip."

So as a boy, when water spurted from my tear ducts because I was sad or upset about something, dad would say, "If you're going to cry, I'll give you something to cry about!" That effectively tabooed crying. So in our home, crying and expressing anything that could be read as "weakness" were *the forbidden emotions* above all others. So I learned to avoid crying, I suppressed crying, and I refused to allow crying in myself and others.

So when it happened that I felt a strong sense of loss and grief as a twenty-three year old, voices arose in my head warning and screaming. They forbid that I would so much as shed a tear or allow the feeling of sadness. "You'll be a sissy! They'll take advantage of you! You'll look foolish and silly!"

Prior to that event, none of this was conscious, but at twenty-three, perhaps for the first time in my life, I actually became *aware* of this. And, as I did, I also simultaneously became aware of how ridiculous it all was. So I did a startlingly shocking thing. I quieted myself and then, just inside my own mind, I said, "I give myself permission to be sad, to feel this loss, and to cry."

Of course, that activated the prohibition frame and all of the sick meanings that I had both received and created about sadness. The dragons were raging and breathing fire, threatening that it would be the end of me and the end of life as I knew it. "You'll be a sissy! You'll be a wimp! Nobody will want to be around you."

It was on that day that I first began creating a *Crucible* of acceptance and acknowledgment for the tabooed emotion of sadness. And with that acceptance, the most paradoxical thing happened. Welcoming that which had been so terrifying actually made me more free, more open, more able to cope, more self-accepting, more accepting of reality as it is, and therefore more realistic and able to cope with losses.

Crucible Coaching
In your notebook, *My Transformational Life,* devote a page to "Emotions." And begin by making your list of emotions that you need a better relationship with. As you observe your emotions and emotional reactions in the next week or two, identify those that you want more control over.

Now that you have a pattern that you can use to reframe all of your emotions, The Meta-Stating Negative Emotions pattern, take time this week to set new frames around the emotion that gives you difficulty. You'll know that you have succeeded when just thinking about that emotion leaves you in a neutral state. It ceases to push your buttons.

Emotions are just emotions and not commands from heaven. Emotions are also symptomatic of many other things—your general sense of health, your belief frames about emotions, and your basic coping skills and competencies. So are you ready to master your emotions rather than let them master you?

End Notes
1. This chapter comes directly from the book *Unleashed!*, Chapter 9

2. *Coaching Conversations: Meta-Coaching, Volume II* (2004), chapter 15, The Fierce Conversation.

3. We use the term "dragon" and the phrase "Dragon Slaying" in Neuro-Semantics as a metaphor for *unresourceful states*. See *Dragon Slaying and Taming* (2000).

4. There are several other patterns in Neuro-Semantics for creating a Crucible of acceptance, the Releasing Judgment pattern, the Accepting, Appreciating, and Esteeming of Self pattern.

5. I quoted this in *Emotions: Sometimes I Have Them/ Sometimes They Have Me* (1985, pages 213-214).

Chapter 6

EVERYDAY CRUCIBLES

Using Life's Challenges, Disappointments, and Traumas as Crucibles for Change

"Tragedy is different from other life situations because it takes us out of the *Deficiency-realm* and into the *Being realm*. That is, tragedy confronts us with the ultimate values, questions, and problems that we ordinarily forget about in everyday existence. With tragedy, we live on the highest plane." Abraham Maslow (1996, p. 56)

Is life a crucible? Has it been for you? Could it be? To actualize your highest and best, you have to encounter yourself to "know thyself," to discover your talents, your likes and dislikes. And all of this requires that you *go through a very personal encounter* in the fires of transformation, the fires of creation.

I didn't know that when I first began studying and researching self-actualization. That discovery came along the way. When I began I didn't understand what a Crucible would be for or why it would be necessary. These are things I have learned along the way.
- What's involved in going through the fires of change?
- How can you transform disruptive experiences in life so they work as a transformative Crucible?
- How can you become a living human Crucible for another person?

The Crucible as a Metaphor

I have been using the image of a *crucible* intentionally to speak about transformational change. In the physical world, we use a crucible to melt down alloys and pour the bubbling, boiling metal into a container so that when it cools, the metal will have a new form and use. We use crucibles to achieve this. And as already noted, it is fascinating that crucibles are typically made out of fairly fragile materials so that if you dropped one on a concrete floor, it would crack or possibly shatter. Fragile in itself, yet a crucible holds the heat and intensity of the temperature of the metal to give it a new shape, to transform the metal.

Maslow argued that *crucible experiences* occur in the process of self-actualization as you unleash and actualize your potentials. *Why is this? How does this work?*

First, the why question. The reason why is because in actualizing your potentials you will, on occasion, need to melt down old forms of thinking, emoting, and behaving in order to mold them into new forms. That's where the Crucible comes in. To become your best version of you, you will need the dross of life, experiences, and mind, burned away. At times, that which is a potentiality will only emerge after you have melted down some of your current habits and styles of thinking, emoting, speaking, and acting. That is, often what holds you back and interferes with releasing some potential new skill or competency is a current habit or form of life.

What is first needed is a context where you can use some pressure or stress that turns up the temperature on your thinking and feeling. In that context you can then let your old forms melt, or burn away, and experience the disintegration of your current forms of thinking-emoting. Then you can hold the space so that a new form and mold can receive all of the raw intensity of your needs, drives, passions, fears, etc.
- So what makes up this context, this space?
- What creates a human crucible?
- How many kinds of crucibles are there?
- How can we consciously create a crucible for transformation?

Naturally Occurring Crucibles

Crucibles for transformation and self-actualization actually occur naturally in life. Such crucibles can entail a wide range of things. They often involve a challenging situation and the pressure that you experienced when you set some outrageous goal that you went for. They can occur with a probing question that opens up unexplored territory within you. Or, they can involve a terrifying problem, a life-threatening illness, a significant loss or disruption in life.[1]

Any of these experiences can become a crucible—a place where the fires of transformation burn off what has been to create space for something that can be. When this happens the experience becomes a very special space for you. It becomes a space where the form of your energies can be taken apart and put back together to create new forms. In this space, you "get to the heart of things" where you then experience a transformation of your thinking, emoting, dreaming, relating, and self-actualizing. No wonder a human Crucible is a very special event and one that you typically dread and fear. It is simultaneously awful and it is awe-ful!

Intentionally Constructing a Crucible

I've been describing how to create a human Crucible—one where you can manage its power so it doesn't put you off in fear or anxiety. So you don't have to wait for some experience that threatens your way of life. You can take charge of the experience and use it intentionally as a transformative process. So as we have learned to tame fire and to use it for cooking, warmth, energy, etc., so we can also tame the fires of human creation and transformation.

With this metaphor in mind, consider how *training* and *coaching* can (if handled properly) operate as crucible experiences. In each of these, there is a person who has certain expert knowledge and skill to support a particular human transformation. An effective trainer or coach is also a person who is equipped to *create a crucible space and hold it* for their clients or participants.

What is this special space? How do we describe it? To describe it I will speak about the three stages that are involved in the process of experiencing the Crucible.

Stage I: The Context of Safety

The first stage is characterized by *awareness, acceptance, and esteem.* These states are designed so that you will feel safe enough to *be*, to be real, and to live with the rough and tumble of your own authenticity. This safety also arises from the trainer or coach's belief in you—in your potential to learn and to become so much more than you are. Once there is safety and the permission to explore, to learn, to be curious, to let things emerge, into the space you are able to bring an openness to the unknown and the unexpected. This prepares you for change. Your awareness is to be *present* to what *is* and to exercise the ego-strength to face reality as it is.

Stage II: The Encounter of Truth
With the safety to change that comes from sufficient ego-strength, unconditional positive regard, non-judgmental awareness, and acceptance, you now have the conditions whereby you can now face the truth of your life—your personal truths. First you adopt a ruthless honesty so you are able to tell yourself the truth. This enables you to face whatever is the case in reality without blinking, without caving in, without escaping, and without putting up ego-defenses. Your truth can then be like a fire, a purging, cleansing truth—the fire of truth, of reality, and of authenticity which heats up the Crucible.

This explains why it takes a highly trained facilitator to create and hold such a space. It takes a person who knows how to elicit and build up a person's ego strength and then invite that person to courageously step up to become all that he or she can become. Ideally, that person has faced his or her own fears of growth and greatness.

In the relational context of being in someone's presence who will not let you off the hook, who passionately believes in you and your possibilities, and who is committed to your growth, *the heat and intensity of the conversation* that arises is what enables you to get to the heart of things where you can experience surprising transformations. That's why it is the fierce conversation that usually facilitates getting to the heart of things. It's a conversation that holds your feet to the fire of creativity and renewal.

The power of the Crucible is that here your hot thoughts can bubble up and then the old experiences can melt so that you can reconstitute them. It is in the melting down of your mental and emotional structures that allows you to form something new, something useful, and something valuable.

After honesty comes *appreciation.* This is the ability to see value, embrace value, and to cling to what's valuable as you simultaneously release dis-values. By bringing the heat of your experiences (your emotions, needs, impulses, drives, thoughts, hopes, fears, etc.) into the Crucible you encounter it with truth. But truth alone is not enough, you also need to encounter it with *appreciation.* You encounter it with value, with positive and rich meaning-making. And when you encounter it with these things, you are able to sacrilize your world.

You also encounter it with *responsibility.* What you find as truths that you speak to yourself and truths about value and meaning, you then take ownership. You move to the point of choice where you make an executive decision about what to do with it, what to embrace as a value and truth to keep with you, and what to release and let go.

Stage III   The Consequence
The third and final stage occurs as you leave the Crucible. It occurs as a consequence of your truth-telling encounter that you appreciate and own. Here you experience *love* or *passion* or *joy* or *ecstasy* as the new expressions begin to emerge from the melt-down in the Crucible. It is not enough to merely dissolve old issues, interpretations, and meanings. You must let the impulses, drives, needs, emotions, thoughts, meanings, etc. reform so that you develop and create new expressions.

The questions that can let you know that you have arrived at this stage include the following:
> "What are you falling in love with? What joy is arising within you? What new passions have emerged or are emerging that you can give yourself to as a valued option?"

It is the passion of falling in love with life and with a specific engagement that brings the feel of self-actualization as you reflect upon it—delight, joy, humor, creativity, etc.

Experiencing the Crucible Experience
A human Crucible is the sacred space created for you by a trainer, a coach, a mentor, a consultant, a friend, a parent, someone who is skilled enough to not be afraid of human stuff (emotions, needs, fears, dreams, passions, greatness, desperation, etc.) and who will be with you, stand by you, and not let you off the hook. Yet of all of these professions, *coaching* is the one that most completely operates as a Crucible.

I say that because, unlike the other professions which has their own expertise and invested interests, *coaching is strictly a meta-discipline that specializes in process expertise, not in content expertise.* The coach enters the human relationship context without a single agenda except to facilitate from the client his or her goals, resources, dreams, fears, potentials, talents, and to hold the space with questioning, accountability, and intensity of reflection and feedback to facilitate a transformation.

This can also happen in trainings—if the training is well designed and well executed. In that situation, the specific information content of the training provides the new learnings to be incorporated and actualized. The transformations are related to the training context. The training then becomes a Crucible in service of that content. Then the various challenges, drills, and practices *comprise and hold the space* where you can play and experiment until the learnings become embodied.

In these instances, the trainer or coach set out to create a controlled and highly managed context as a *human Crucible* with the design of personality change and life transformation. As such, that's what a client or a training participant pays for. That's why we search out top-notch trainers, consultants, and coaches and put ourselves into those contexts so as to guide and direct the discipline of the transformation.

When Life's Challenges become a Crucible
But do you have to engage a professional coach, trainer, consultant, etc.? Yes and no. While life can be a crucible, and while we can intentionally create an interpersonal space in training and coaching for a crucible, to put such experiences to good use as a transformative Crucible, you have to bring intentionality, acceptance, courage, and understanding to your life experience. Failure to put these experiences to good use explains why most people do not get much from these experiences or challenges.

This premise about adult learning, growing, and self-actualizing raises crucial questions:
- How can you use your events, relationships, trials, and experiences as a crucible of transformation?
- How can you use life's experiences as a resource for transformation?
- How can you enter into the fire of creation to invent new ways of being using some life experience that was a real challenge to you?

Typically when a challenge or threat arises, it is unplanned. And that's why you typically feel out of control. This is the key difference between life's experiences and those planned experiences in trainings, coaching, apprenticeships, etc. In life it just happens. It happens without your choice, desire, or planning. And so you mostly experience it *reactively*—you react to the turns and twists of life, to the ups-and-downs of work, relationships, health, economics, etc. And so no wonder most of us feel that experience as a crucible as unpleasant, painful, destructive, and to be avoided at all costs. Isn't that true for you? Do you have an undigested experience that's still within you taking up space and energy?

Yet experience per se does not guarantee transformation. An experience in itself does not guarantee positive, passionate, and highly desired transformations. Problems, challenges, disappointments, upsets, etc. are just as likely to make you bitter as better. The difference, of course, is your attitude—which comes from the meanings you give the experience. The difference is how you take, handle, and explain the experience. Here *your explanatory style,* will determine whether you use the experience for transformation or not. Here everything comes down to meaning—to your ability to create meaning, to enter the Crucible, release old meanings and construct new ones.

Enabling a Crucible Experience

If every experience is not a crucible, what enables some experiences to become a Crucible of transformation for you? More likely than not, you will not naturally and easily utilize the experiences that could become the foundation for transformation. Instead you will avoid using your experiences as crucibles because your natural tendency is to defend against it. You will naturally seek to escape it. In order to allow something that's a problem, that induces negative emotions, pressure, etc. to work as a Crucible—*you have to stay with it and welcome it*. And this may require a complete change of your attitude. You have to do what is so counter-intuitive—to *accept it* and *look for value in it*.
- So what enables you to transform an experience into a positive transformative one?
- How can you turn your experiences into crucibles of change?

Prerequisites for a Human Crucible

For an experience to become a crucible, it needs to meet several conditions. Minimally, it needs to have the capacity to hold three things:
1) Heat
2) Time-Space
3) Ownership of Meaning

1) Heat: *The experience has to activate and hold an intensity of emotion and energy.*
Not everything that happens to you or that you experience is capable of being a Crucible, only those things that activate sufficient energy in your needs, drives, emotions, thoughts, hopes, dreams, fears, appreciations, etc. What will do that? Threats, problems, pressures, stresses, challenges, confusions, wonder, falling in love, curiosities, etc.

To be a Crucible, there needs to be enough human energy as heat to melt down your current forms and expressions of life— your current thought patterns, attitudes, ways of emoting, rituals, habits, lifestyles, cultural structures, etc. Typically you will experience this *heat* as stress, pressure, disruptions, disappointments, anger, grief, and confusion. You could, however, just as well experience it as passion, excitement, impatience, joy, anticipation.

What determines sufficient intensity of energy is meaning. Is it meaningful? Is it significant? Does it matter? Does it matter *for* you or *against* you? If not, then insufficient intensity. If yes, then you have the beginnings of a Crucible in the making.

2) Time-Space: *You have to stay inside the experience for a sufficient time.*
While a short experience that happens and is over quickly could be a Crucible, it has to have an enormous amount of intensity, a level that is usually traumatic or life changing in impact. Yet when that happens you are more likely than not to feel overwhelmed which explains why you won't use it for transformation, at least most of us don't.

More typically, Crucible experiences will involve an experience that lasts for days, weeks, even years. It has to last long enough so that its heat causes you to melt down. It goes on long enough that your traditional and habitual ways of operating, thinking, feeling, relating, etc. no longer work. And it is in that ineffectiveness of your current ways that moves you to look around and to try something else. This is the unfreezing of the old pattern before the creation of the new.

What is required for staying with an experience? You have to choose to be present with something, to welcome it into your consciousness, emotions, and life to adjust and adapt to it. To then reflect upon it and to give it your full presence and mindfulness.

That's why it is the experience that won't let you escape or defend against it and that forces you to face your current forms that gives you a chance to re-mold them. This typically happens when you have a big and bold enough of a goal that keeps you in something for a month or a year— an adventure, an job, a career, a committed relationship, a sports season, etc. Or when someone holds the space and won't let you avoid or run away from it.

3) *Ownership of Meaning:* *You have to use the experience for transformation.*
For the experience to evoke, elicit, and provoke change in you, as you are *with* the experience, you experience a melt-down, a releasing of the old, a questioning of the old, an explanation of the new. Now while an overwhelming experience may cause a "melt down," you may not put the melt down to creative and positive use unless you have a sense that you can direct and guide the new forms. This is where acceptance gives you that kind of control.

Best is an experience that keeps the pressure on, that keeps challenging you and does so just a little bit beyond your current skills and understandings. Then instead of crushing your spirit, you keep resiliently coming back and stretching and accessing potential resources you never knew you had. This requires resilience and a solution-focus orientation of looking for resources for coping and developing problem-solving skills.

Unless there is inner change that you own as yours, the experience will not be positively transformational. That's why any experience that's overwhelming generally does not result in positive change.

The experience has to have sufficient pressure to reveal, create, and develop your character, but not too much. And within the experience there must still be an awareness that you'll get through it, you will survive, and you will conquer it. You have to maintain hope and courage. You have to keep calling to your depths and reaching within to access resources you had no awareness are there. Often this happens with people you meet along the way who encourage you and who stand by you. Sometimes it happens when you meet someone in a book or story or film who serves as your mentor and coach.

Bringing it altogether

While it's possible to do this by yourself, I don't recommend it. While heroic figures arise from time to time who are able to re-invent themselves, and allow that experience to be like a Crucible so that it melts down life and gave space for new frames to emerge, going it alone takes a lot longer. And it is usually a lot harder. It means spending much more time in "the dark night of the soul," and it usually involves lots of unnecessary pain and emotional distress. Viktor Frankl did it alone and out of it created Logo-Therapy, but he was in prison and didn't have much choice.

We really do need each other. It is so much more effective to experience transformation when there is someone who will go with you and be with you providing the context and Crucible space. Ultimately that is what training, apprenticeships, mentoring relationships, and especially coaching offers. In Meta-Coaching, we train our coaches to become the kind of persons who can "hold the space" with acceptance, non-intrusive witnessing, care and respect, and then bold, ruthless questioning so that they can quickly enable a person to "get to the heart of things."

We call this the *dance of change* and use *the Axes of Change* to facilitate the process, and we do so in such a way that the crucible experience becomes not only a highly valued one, but also one that's more fun and playful than painful and disruptive. And that occurs because our coaches also know how to empower the ego-strength of clients so as to take full ownership of their creative meaning-making. The result is a transformation not only of specific life changes, but of one's relationship to change — so that we become change-embracers, resilient change-embracers who are thinking ahead about new challenges and potentials to unleash and who don't fear the process at all but embrace it as the path of self-actualization.

Crucible Coaching

In your notebook, *My Transformational Life,* make a page that you devote to "Natural Crucibles." If life itself is full of naturally occurring Crucibles, what crucibles have you experienced in life? Make a list.

Once you have your list, revisit those crucible experiences with the following questions:
- Were you safe enough in that crucible experience to put it to good use?
- Were you able to witness it and accept it?

Was your value and worth as a person at stake in that crucible?
What truth, responsibility, or appreciation were you able to discover in that crucible?

If you were not ready with the transformational resources for handling the natural life crucible, then consider whether it would be valuable to revisit that life experience now and take into your Crucible. If so, then if you can do it by yourself, then do so. Or if you need someone to facilitate the process, then find someone to do that.

In NLP we say, "It is never too late to have a happy childhood." We say that because the memory you carry around with you is *your* memory— a *construct that you have created and continue to create.* So what have you constructed about old experiences? Does it support you and your self-actualization? Does it empower you or diminish you? What happened is one thing, *how you remember it and how you use it* is an entirely different one.

End of the Chapter References
1. See *Unleashed!* (2007). Chapter 20, "Capitalizing Problems."

PART II

CRUCIBLE

ELEMENTS

Chapter 7

UNCONDITIONAL POSITIVE REGARD

You are Not the Problem!

> "No psychological health is possible
> unless the essential core of the person
> is fundamentally accepted, loved,
> and respected by others and by himself."
> Abraham Maslow

> "We all want to be recognized and accepted for what we are
> in our fullness, richness, and complexity."
> Abraham Maslow (1968, p. 93)

The very first element for a transformational Crucible is unconditional positive regard for yourself as a human being. Maslow (1968) wrote about the importance of valuing and esteeming the person with unconditional love and acceptance:

> "If humanness is accepted and loved, then many local, ethnocentric problems simply disappear. . . . "No psychological health is possible unless the essential core of the person is fundamentally accepted, loved, and respected." (1968, p. 196)

The philosophy of the Crucible is that it enables you to access and utilize your self-at-your-best (rather than at your worst). It takes you into your highest potentials, not your lowest reactivity. And to do that we start with a radical declaration— *Human nature is good!* In fact, I'll go further. It is not only good, *human nature is special—sacred and should be treated with love and respect.*

Carl Rogers, even more so than Maslow, believed so much in the natural organic nature of change that he argued that anyone helping with it should do so completely in a *non-directive* way. This, in fact, became his brand— non-directive therapy. For him, change under good conditions will inevitably and naturally happen.

> "[Acceptance] seems to me to have value because the curious paradox is that *when I accept myself as I am, then I change.* . . . We cannot change, we cannot move away from what we are, until we thoroughly *accept* what we are. Then change seems to come about almost unnoticed." (Rogers, 1961, p. 17 italics added)

To facilitate this organic nature of change, the therapist (or coach, helper, facilitator, or parent) uses his or her own authenticity and genuine reality. The change-agent works first and foremost on self. Only then are you truly ready to work with others.

> "The more I am simply willing to be myself and the more I am willing to understand and accept the realities in myself and in the other person, the more change seems to be stirred up. It is a very paradoxical thing— that to the degree that each one of us is willing to be himself, then he finds not only himself changing but he finds that other people to whom he relates are also changing." (1961, p. 21)

As you can tell from that quote, for Rogers, *the facilitator's own authenticity and being-ness* is his or her primary tool for facilitating change.

> "Personal change is facilitated when the psychotherapist *is* what he *is,* when in the relationship with his client he is genuine and without 'front' or facade, openly being the feeling and attitudes which at that moment are flowing *in* him. The more genuine and congruent the therapist in the relationship, the more probability there is that change in personality in the client will occur." (1961: 62)

That which creates the "space"—the atmosphere and the context of the Crucible for self-actualizing growth and the unleashing of potentials—is the acceptance, care, concern, and warm regard of the person who holds the space—the Crucible space is loved into existence.

> "The more *acceptance* and *liking* I feel toward this individual, the

> more I will be creating a relationship which he can use. By acceptance I mean *a warm regard* for him as a person of unconditional self-worth—of value no matter what his condition, behavior or feelings. I feel a continuing desire to understand—a sensitive empathy with each of the client's feelings and communications as they seem to him at that moment." (1961: 33)

Something else further creates this special space. It is the belief in the client's potentialities and behaving toward him or her in a way that externalizes that belief.

> "If I accept him [my client] as *a process of becoming,* then I am doing what I can to confirm or make real his potentialities. If I see this as his potentiality, he tends to act in ways which support this hypothesis. If I see a relationship as an opportunity to reinforce *all* that he is, the person that he is with all his existent potentialities, then he tends to act in ways which support *this* hypothesis." (1961: 55, 56)

So for Rogers these were the critical factors that create a crucible for encounter and transformation. Listening empathetically to the person enables that person to begin to learn how to listen to him or herself in a new way—in an accepting way. That cuts out the judgment (the negative evaluation meta-state that creates internal monsters and dragons) and begins to set frames for discovery and understanding. Rogers says it frees the person from rigidity, fixity, and coldness in functioning.

Developing Unconditional Positive Regard

To regard yourself and every other human being with a positive regard that's unconditional is to *esteem the human "self" as unconditionally valuable, precious, mysterious, wonderful, and worthwhile.* And to do this requires that you look at your philosophy and psychology about your "sense of self" in all of its numerous factors: self-esteem, self-confidence, ego, ego-strength, social self, self-image, etc. So if you're ready, let's do that.

First, Distinguish Self-Esteem from Self-Confidence
This is not only the first, it is also the most important step. It is also a step that you will not find in most psychology books. So what's the difference? *Self-esteem* refers to a person's value, worth, dignity, honor, and loveability. It has nothing to do with what you can *do*, what you are good at, your talents, dispositions, gifts, or achievements. Those facets define *self-*

confidence.

As a verb, *esteem* refers to a mental evaluation or judgment. It refers to how you *appraise the value* of something. And, as such, it is based on a criterion or several criteria. But what criterion? When it comes a self-esteem, upon what do you base your evaluation? Is that evaluation conditional or unconditional? If conditional, then upon what conditions? Do you base the evaluation on a person's looks, intelligence, skills, cooperative nature, strength, speed, grades, money, relationships, etc.? Whatever you base the person's value on —that then becomes the self-esteem conditions that you use —consciously or unconsciously.

Self-Esteem

Conditional	——	**Unconditional**
Based on conditions		Based on no conditions
Earned		Recognized as a gift
Always "on the line"		Never in question
Hoping to become a Somebody		Born a Somebody

If you value a person (including yourself) as having value, esteem, worth, dignity, honor, etc., based on any conditions, then you are conditionally valuing that person. You are believing and expecting that *the person has to earn it.* The person has to prove him or herself worthy of the value you attribute. And because the person has to continually earn it, the person is on a treadmill—always trying to prove him or herself. *Conditional* self-esteem implies a person is not okay in and of him or herself, the person has to earn your right to be valued as a person. Now imagine doing that to anyone. Do that to a child and you rob your child of his or her innate right to be an innately valuable human being. And that will set the child up to feel anxious about his or her very existence. You have posited the child's self-worth as "on the line" and liable to be destroyed.

By contrast, *unconditional* self-esteem makes the criterion singular— *if you are a human being, you have innate worth and value.* Your dignity and honor is a given, you were born with dignity. You don't have to prove anything to be seen, recognized, and accepted as a full human being. And if your worth is a given, you don't have to prove anything to be a somebody.

You already are a somebody and now you have the right and freedom to fully express your somebodyness.

Typically most of us confuse self-esteem and self-confidence and speak about these two states as if they are synonyms. They are not. Even psychology books still interchange these words making no distinction between them. They present self-esteem as if it is something conditioned upon a person's feelings of confidence about achievements. Once that assumption is made, then the assumption is that you have to encourage a person to "build up his or her self-esteem" by encouraging the person to find his or her strengths and develop them. Do that to a person and you are subtly suggesting that the person has to "earn" his or her worth as a human being.

A sign of this confusion shows up also in our language every time we speak about *high* or *low* self-esteem. *Yet if self-esteem can be high (or low), then it is conditional.* It can go up or down. And if it is conditional, then not a given. It is not unconditional. Then it can be lost.

> *If you are a human being, you have innate worth and value.* Your dignity and honor is a given, you were born with dignity.

By contrast, if your esteem as a human being is unconditional, then you can *esteem* your worth or value as unquestionable. You attribute to yourself, and everyone else, the honor and dignity of being a *human being* and therefore special, unique, and sacred.

The How of Self-Esteeming
Since this is not how most people think about self-esteem, the questions arise: *How* do we give self-esteem to ourselves, to our children, or to any person? *How* do we distinguish a person's worth and humanness from his or her activities and achievements?

When I became a parent, and especially a single-parent raising a daughter from the age of three by myself, I took special care to make this distinction. Actually it was an easy thing to do—something navigated mostly by language. What I found challenging was to remember this as she grew up and became a teenager (!).

    "You did that really well! I think that's one of your strengths (or gifts). Well done!"

    "Whether you succeed in the gymnastic meet today or not, you are an absolutely valuable and lovable person and nothing can take away from that. So go out there, give it your best; have fun and we'll see what happens."

"Well, I think you know what I'm going to say. Do you? Yes, you shouldn't have done that. And you know what the consequences are—you have to do a time-out in your bedroom. And I want you to know that I love you absolutely!"

Ultimately the answer is not all that difficult or complex if you know *the self-esteem—self-confidence difference.* To do that, think about something that you esteem as having innate worth and value. Do you have anything like that? Have you ever stood in amazement at something, or in awe of something that just *is,* and that doesn't have to *do* anything to be so recognized? Here are some possibilities:

- Holding a newborn baby in your arms and feeling a sense of awe in the value of the child, the mystery of life, the magic of love, the wonder of the baby's humanity?
- Standing in awe of a beautiful sunrise or sunset, recognizing the wonder of the planet circling the sun and spinning around.
- Standing on top of a mountain on a cloudless night and seeing the Milky Way Galaxy and sensing the immensity of the universe.

The feeling of awe arises when you recognize the ultimate sense of esteem, worth, or value. So when you feel *awe*, take a moment to capture that feeling. Be with that feeling. That's the feeling of accepting or acknowledging the value and worth of something for what it *is*. Now, taking that feeling, apply that to yourself and acknowledge that *being* a human being is something that just *is*. Now stand in awe of that mystery, that awesome sacredness of what you are as a human being.

This is the structure of self esteeming. Doing this provides a good model of living from your dignity—an important example for your child. So take that feeling of awe and apply it to the person before you so that you can *stand in awe of that person's innate worth and value* and as you do, *recognize that it is unconditional.* Say to yourself, "This person doesn't have to prove anything or achieve anything to be fully valuable as a person." Declare this as a fact that you simply recognize—everybody *is* a somebody. Period. He or she doesn't have to prove anything, earn anything. Every person you met is an awesome being with incredible possibilities.

The Crucible Chapter 7 *Unconditional Positive Regard*

Second, Appreciate the Person's Powers and Achievements

If that's self-esteem, then *self-confidence* is about your faith with yourself to *do*. The word "confidence" tells the story. *Fideo* is faith or trust which you have "with" (*con*) yourself. You trust or believe in your ability to *do* something. What are you confident about? Typing? Riding a bike? Washing your clothes? Cooking a meal? Reading? Whatever it is, you are confident about a *skill* that you can *perform*. If you have a skill that you are just learning, you probably are not confident about it— yet. But if you keep at it, keep learning, experimenting, receiving feedback, etc., then you will develop the feeling of confidence regarding that skill.

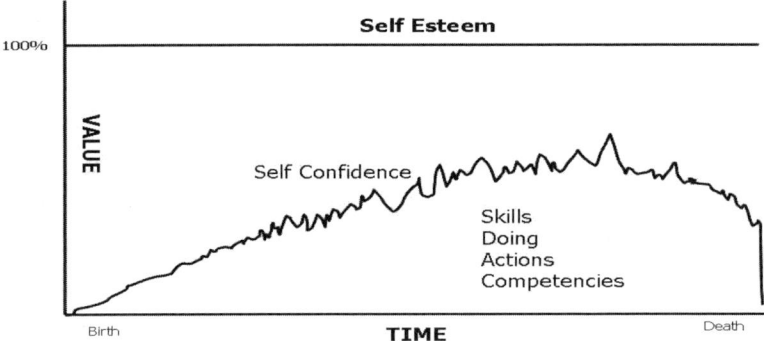

Unlike self-esteem, *self-confidence is conditional.* You have to earn it. You have to prove that you can actually *do* the thing that you're confident about.

If you are a parent or a lover, or a leader, manager, consultant, or coach, be careful to not make the other's sense of self-value *conditioned* on his or her skills, gifts, strengths, or successes. Yes, value them, appreciate them, and esteem their skills and achievements, but *don't connect these things or experiences to making the person a better person or a "somebody."* It does not. Sure, the accomplishments will influence his or her self-confidence, and it should. But don't link it to his or her value as a human being. It does not make the person one iota of a more valuable person.

> "You are really good at music (or whatever). You have an ear for it! That's good, maybe you would like to learn to play an instrument or join the choir."

The backside of this is enabling your child, friend, lover, employee to accept and to live comfortably with the areas in which he or she is not naturally talented:

> "While you are really good at mathematics, your gifts make you different from your brother who is really good at music. It's okay. Now you can focus your interest on your talent and potentials. Isn't that great?"

Contrastive Difference Between	
Self-Esteem	**Self-Confidence**
About being-ness	About talents and skills
Human Being	Human Doing
Being as a person	Doing as an achiever
Unconditional	Conditional
Don't have to prove	Must prove yourself
Realm of "person"	Realm of competency and achievement
Be in order to do	Do in order to achieve
Value of your person	Trust in what you can do

The person who demands the feeling of confidence in something *prior* to learning is requiring either the impossible or is drowning in a fool's desire. I say "the impossible" because to have confidence in yourself that you can do something *before* you do it is by definition —impossible or stupid. And I say "a fool's desire" because *if* you did access a feeling of confidence regarding something in which you are actually incompetent, then that feeling of confidence would only make you a fool. You would *feel* that you could do something when you cannot! We have a name for people like that—"fools."

Begin by distinguishing person and behavior. Embody this knowing at the feeling level that people are more than their actions. Know this about yourself; *you are more than your behaviors.* You are more than your thoughts, your emotions, your responses. How well do you know this about yourself?

This realization of the difference between person and behavior empowers you to *unconditionally* value and esteem yourself as "somebody" so that you do not put your value on the line based on some fallible aspect of human nature, like your thinking, feeling, acting, understanding, etc. And when you can do that with yourself, you can do the same with others. When you deal with people, you deal with their expressions of thoughts, feelings, speech and behavior—not them as a person. Their person remains a mystery—a sacred mystery.

Moving from Self-Confidence to Self-Efficacy
Once you develop confidence in one thing, and then another, and then many others, eventually another state can emerge. When you develop self-confidence once and again in a variety of areas, it means that you have repeatedly moved from incompetence to competence. It means you have learned and developed one particular skill, and then another. And at first, it always seems so impossible. Hard. But eventually, you realize that it is just the learning process. And with that, *self-efficacy* begins.

What's the difference? Self-confidence relates to the past—to the skills that you have already developed. *Your confidence in what you can do has proof.* You have evidence for your confidence. It's credible. You know you can do something because you have done it before and you have done it often enough that you now trust yourself, and now feel convinced that you can do it again and again. You can perform it on demand.
Self-efficacy relates to the future and to the skills that you will develop, or even could develop, if you so choose. Your sense of confidence in those yet-to-be-developed skills of the future has no historical proof, no evidence that you can point to and say, "See I have done that before!" Instead what convinces you is something else, it is your sense of confidence in *you*, in your ability to learn, to develop, to walk through the learning process. It is your sense of confidence that you can trust your wits, your intelligence, your emotions, your ability to relate to others, and so on. That's self-efficacy.

As an example, I have a sense of self-confidence in driving a car. I've been driving since I was 16 and have driven without an accident of any sort for over 30 years. Further, I have driven in countries that drive on the right side of the road (in the USA) and the left side (in Australia). I have lots of history that can booster up my confidence about driving a car. But since I have never flown a plane, I do not have confidence about doing that. But I have a sense of self-efficacy that *I could* fly a plane in the near future *if I so chose*. Why? How? Because I know that it's just a matter of learning and practice. I know that I could sign up for a course or get a private tutor to guide me through the process. I know of many friends who have their pilot's license and I could speak with them about the process.

It is self-efficacy, rather than self-confidence, that gives you a sense of taking on the world and following your dreams. Eventually you learn that the early stage of not-knowing something and feeling incompetent in a new area, and sometimes even overwhelmed—all of that is just *part of the process of becoming competent.* There's no need to misread or over-load the confusion or disorientation with negative meanings. It is the process everybody goes through in developing competence and then mastery.[2]

Fourth, Enable the Development of a Strong Ego.
"Ego" is simply a Greek word for "self," "I" and/or "me." It is the very word used in the Greek New Testament every time Jesus said "I am the good shepherd," or "I am the vine." There's nothing wrong with "ego" or having an ego. Every thinking person who can face reality has an "ego." For Sigmund Freud, *ego* refers to "the reality principle" and so to the ability to face reality for what it is.

Contrastive Difference Between

Self-Confidence ——>	Self-Efficacy
Able to *do* something Development of a *skill* able to *achieve* action or experience	Not able to do something *yet* trust in oneself that I will be able to develop the new skill or competence.
From incompetence to competence and then to expertise.	Realization: I have developed many competencies and that means I can trust my future abilities and potentials.
Proof from the past	Trust in the future.

As a sense of self, no one is born with an "ego." At first, a newborn infant is undifferentiated from mother. Then ever so slowly, the infant begins to discover itself to be a self, one separate from mother. And this differentiation and individuation continues until the young child knows him or herself as a separate person.

So ego-strength is the strength of your sense of self to look at what *is* in the face without falling apart, caving in, or having some fight or flight response.

No one is born with this, it develops. It develops as you develop a sense of your value and your confidence in your skills. It especially develops as you develop effective skills in coping with your basic needs and drives.

Ego-strength is a consequence of discovering and developing your four innate powers—your mental powers, emotional powers, verbal and linguistic powers, and powers of action. These four powers enable you to feel in control of yourself—your mind, emotions, and verbal and behavioral responses. And this creates a sense of empowerment and response-ability.

The sense of ownership emerges in children very early, in the second year. That's when they first learn to word, "mine." This isn't a sign of selfishness. It is a sign of development of personality, of taking ownership and responsibility. As the child welcomes things, experiences, and people into her world, she becomes richer within herself. If you don't demonize this, you can help your child develop his sense of ownership for his thoughts, emotions, words, and actions —the key variables for responsibility and proactivity.

Meta-Stating Your "Self" Pattern
The following pattern is the most basic meta-state process for inducing three basic *self* states: self-acceptance, self-appreciation, and self-esteem! Use it to establish a solid core for centering yourself for setting a frame of high value and worth for oneself, and for operating with high self-esteem even in the face of dignity-denying or threatening experiences. I have put three states (acceptance, appreciation, and awe) on the continuum of *liking* and *welcoming* something into your world.

Rejection	*Acceptance*	*Appreciation*	*Esteem*
Dislike	Welcoming — Inviting in	Gentle openness	High valuing as important
Judgment	Non-Judgment	Welcome warmly	Significant, worthwhile
Rejection	w/o endorsement Acknowledge but no condoning or endorsing	with attraction / love	Welcome with Awe, Honor
		— **Doing** —	**Being / Person**

The key distinction you will be making as you use this pattern is the distinction between self-esteem as unconditional (based on an evaluation or judgment of the mind) and self-confidence as conditional (based on competency and experience). The situations that you can use this pattern can be elicited by the following questions: Do you ever judge your self as a human being? Do you ever put yourself down? Contempt yourself? Insult yourself? Do you have conditional self-esteem? Do you separate your feelings about you as a human being from your feelings as a human doing? If yes, then by all means, use the following pattern.

Meta-Stating Self Pattern[3]
1) Access each of the three states — Acceptance, Appreciation, and Awe.
Access each state by using a small and simple referent so that you can access the feeling of the state fully and discreetly.
A) *Acceptance*:
> What do you accept that you could reject? What small and simple thing do you easily accept without particularly liking or wanting, but you welcome? Once you may have hated it, rejected it, got yourself upset about it, but now you find that things go better by just accepting it. A menu list for *acceptance* includes accepting when it's raining, the traffic, taking out the garbage, putting up with noise at the coffee shop, etc.
> [Note: Acceptance is not resignation nor is it condoning. It is acknowledging what *is* as that which exists and has to be dealt with for what it is. Acceptance is typically a very small and gentle feeling in the body. Notice your breath, posture, face, eyes, etc. when you are in that state.]

B) *Appreciation.*
> Is there anything that you really appreciate? What do you really value and appreciate that causes you melt in appreciation? A menu list: holding a newborn baby, watching a beautiful sunset, having a glass of wine with a friend, a back rub, walking on a beach with a loved one, playing with puppies, etc.
> [Appreciation goes far beyond acceptance as it warmly welcomes the valued object. Appreciation is the most emotional of these three states and most easily experienced in the body.]

C) *Awe.*
> What is so big, so wonderful, so marvelous, so incredible that you

stand in awe of it, speechless, in utter wonder? As a menu list consider: standing in the presence of one of the "Wonders of the World," being present at the birth of your child, seeing the Milky Way Galaxy on the top of a mountain, contemplating your understanding of the spiritual, etc.

[Awe, by its very nature, is much less emotional and sometimes involves the feeling of being speechless, beyond words, a state in which you may hold your breath and hardly move as your contemplation tries to take in the greatness of what you are in awe of.]

3) *Amplify each state and apply to yourself [or to the person you are working with].*

As you feel X [acceptance, appreciation, awe], how strong is that feeling? [From 0 to 10.] Now let that feeling grow, let it become stronger and stronger. Double the intensity of that feeling. Let it permeate throughout your body and radiate out. Do you now have a good robust state of X? Anchor the state with a gesture and/or a touch, that is, *link* or *associate* a gesture or a touch to the experience of that state so that it becomes associated with the state.[4]

Now one state at a time, apply the resource to yourself:

Apply acceptance to the things about yourself that you need to accept, but may find challenging to accept— your shadow side, experiences that have happened to you, the cards that life dealt you. Accept your overall sense of self and life.
>
> What do you want to accept?
> What have you spent a lot of time fighting and rejecting that you now know that you need to just accept?
> As you think about that, *feel this* [fire the trigger for acceptance].

Apply appreciation to your sense of self as doer and achiever. Appreciate your over-all self, and every gift, talent, and strength. Feel this sense of *appreciation* to your mind, your emotions, your speech, your behavior.
>
> [This separates self-confidence and self-esteem.]
> What can you appreciate? What else?
> What strengths about yourself do you appreciate?
> As you *feel this*, notice what else you can appreciate.

> *Apply awe and esteem* to your self as a valuable, precious, magnificent human being unconditionally.
> [Use self-esteem to enrich self-appreciation and self-acceptance.]
> > *Feeling this self-esteem* fully and completely, letting it grow and expand ... that's right, now notice what else you can *appreciate* [fire anchor] and what else you can just *accept* [fire anchor] more gracefully and easily. That's right.

4) Apply self-esteeming, appreciating, and accepting to the needed contexts in your life.

> Is there any context, situation, or event wherein you feel tempted to self-contempt, self-question, self-doubt, and/or self-dislike yourself?
>
> In what context do you want to operate from with a solid sense of your unconditional self-esteem?
> As you think about that, *feel this esteem* [fire anchor] for yourself knowing that your worth and value is a given and *feel this appreciation* for what you can do so that you focus there, and *feel this acceptance* of the things that just are that you have to deal with.
>
> Now especially notice how *feeling this esteem and self-awe* at the mystery of you and your potentials transforms this old context. How is that?
> Do you like that? Would that make a difference?
> Are you ready to self-respect yourself no matter what?
> Are you ready to step into unconditional self-esteem?

5) Imaginatively put this solid sense of your self into your future to validate.

> Imagine moving through life in the weeks and months to come with this frame of mind of self-acceptance, self-appreciation, and self-esteem. . . . Do you like this?
> Notice how this would transform things for you . . .
> Does every aspect of the higher parts of your mind fully agree with this?
> Is your sense of your own value now completely set?

Becoming a Human Crucible
To become a living, breathing, and caring human Crucible for yourself or others requires several things. It requires that you distinguish person and

behavior, accept the person, and take second position to empathetically understand the person's inner world. Yet while the Crucible of transformation starts here, it doesn't end here. There's more to a transformative human Crucible, things that Rogers missed.

You can use *the Crucible Model* in a transformational way when you use it to facilitate a person's self-acceptance. Then you can hold a crucial conversation in the Crucible with yourself or another and for the purpose of unleashing potentials.

Your Crucible Conversation
How do you language this distinction when you invite someone into the Crucible? What are the linguistic expressions for unconditional positive regard? Here are some questions you can ask:
- How do you best like to represent that you are more than and different from your actions?
- What will help you to separate your person from your behavior?
- Where in your Crucible space do you want to put this distinction? As you do, what does it look and sound like?
- Do you need a menu list to give these ideas about how to represent this? You could have a sphere of energy representing your "spark of divinity" or "spark of humanness" (your spirit) that you step in and then out of into the world of actions and activities (your body). You could have a floating cloud for your *beingness* and the ground for your *doing*.

Crucible Coaching
It's coaching time! So as you get your notebook, *My Transformational Life*. Title the new page, "Unconditional Positive Regard: Self-Esteem." Now as you review this chapter, make a list of the insights that you have gained.
> How well do you understand the distinction between person and behavior? Do you have full permission within yourself to esteem yourself with unconditional positive value and worth? Get a friend and run the self-acceptance, self-appreciation, and self-esteem pattern. Do that until any thought of self-contempting creates a sense of aversion so that it totally doesn't fit for you.

The ability and attitude of regarding people with positive regard is the beginning, but in itself is not sufficient. The regard must be *unconditional* or you will be applying your evaluations as you judge whether the person measures up to your standards and criteria. Do that, and the person will feel on the defense.

End Notes

1. This pattern is taught in the APG workshops around the world, see the APG Schedule on www.neurosemantics.com.

2. See the book, *Achieving Peak Performance* (2009). The whole book is on the subject of taking effective action and mind-to-muscling what you know so that it is in ready access in your body and available when you need it.

3. For more about the Meta-States model and the process of meta-stating, see *Secrets of Personal Mastery* (1999), *Meta-States* (2007), or *Winning the Inner Game* (2007).

4. "Anchoring" is a process in NLP for linking or associating one thing with another. As such, it is a user-friendly version of conditioning in Behaviorism. The process is described in most introduction books to NLP or you can find it in *Sourcebook of Magic* (1997) or in *User's Manual of the Brain, Volume I* (1999).

Chapter 8

WITNESSING

Pure Attention to What *Is*

"My aim has been to provide a *climate* which contains as much of safety, of warmth, empathetic understanding, as I can genuinely find in myself to give. Away from facades: move away from a self that one is not. Away from oughts. Away from meeting expectations, from the enormous pressures to become the characteristics expected. Away from pleasing others. Toward self-direction: becoming responsible for oneself, deciding what activities and ways of behaving having meaning for you, and what do not. Toward being process: fluidity, changing. An existing individual is constantly in process of becoming."
   Carl Rogers (1961, p. 167)

Once you enter the Crucible space fully recognizing your unconditional value, and that your fallible expressions and experiences are a very different thing, you realize that awareness is your first transformative resource. This is not just any with awareness, it is a special one—pure, simple, sensory awareness. *It is pure and simple because it is being aware without judging.* This requires the ability to see and hear and simply witness what is. Carl Rogers himself did not use the metaphor of a crucible, instead as indicated in the quote at the beginning of this chapter, he spoke of *a climate* that facilitates such awareness.

Now Maslow noted that *whole-hearted attending* to what exists before us is as rare an experience as it is a wearing experience (1970, p. 204). "Wearing" because it requires a lot from you. What does it require and how can you develop pure awareness of what is? How can you step into the transformative state of just witnessing? Here I have listed four essential steps.

Pure Awareness
1) Access Pure Awareness by losing your mind and come to your senses.
2) Move beyond cutting up the world to experience it by stop dichotomizing.
3) Be with what *is* by giving up demanding expectations.
4) Embrace and release your censors by freely associating.

---

1) Lose your mind and come to your senses
On the other hand, *Fritz Perls* (1971) wrote extensively about awareness and especially the special kind of awareness that's required:
> "Without awareness, there is no cognition of choice. Awareness, contact, and being present are merely different aspect of one and the same process—self-realization." (p. 66)
> "Say, 'Now I am aware.' The *now* keeps us in the present and brings home the fact that no experience is ever possible except in the present. The 'I' develops the person's sense of responsibility for his feelings." (p. 65)

Perls refers here to *pure sensory awareness*. Sensory awareness is the awareness that occurs when you can *see-and -see*. It occurs when you can *hear and hear; feel and feel, sense and sense*. That is, you experience the sensory awareness of what *is* for what it is in terms of the sensory information without introjecting any of your ideas, interpretations, or evaluations about it. For Perls, sensory awareness is *contact* with what *is* in the *present* moment without contaminating it with any of your mental models, understandings, or beliefs. The contrast is evaluative awareness—this describes being aware of something through your beliefs, indeed through layers of beliefs in the higher levels of your mind.
> "If you live in the present, you use whatever is available. If you live in your computer or in your thinking machine, or in these obsolete responses or in your rigid way of coping with life, you stay stuck." (Fritz Perls, *Witness to Therapy*, p. 28)

The quotation taken up in NLP that most powerfully expresses this is the classic quotation by Perls:
> *"Lose your mind and come to your senses."*

Consider this radical and humorous statement about "losing your mind." It is an attention-getting call to witness purely what *is*. And to do that requires that you lose you all of the bias and prejudices and beliefs in your meta-mind. Now you just have your sensory-based mind left to be aware of what is. Another awareness that contrasts with this is *synesthesia awareness*. This occurs when you see-and-feel, or hear-and-feel which is a common way that most of us commonly experience our awareness. We see blood and feel fear; or we hear a harsh tonality of voice and feel scolded or threatened. The sight is not just the sight, the sound is not just the sound.

2) Stop Dichotomizing with an Integrative Perspective.

To dichotomize is to think, treat, and impose upon reality either-or opposites as a template. It is to think of opposites, alternatives, and differences and to frame, something as a choice between polarities. So for example,

> **Dichotomy; Dichotomize:** Division, dividing into two parts.

with regard to consciousness dichotomizing means you separate "mind" from "emotion" and treat each as polar opposites, rather than a holistic mind-emotion. Of course, separating what is a whole into parts to do that distorts your sense of what is and prevents you from encountering it as it is.

Attending to what *is* stands in contrast to *rubricizing* reality. This was the word that Maslow most often used. He talked about creating false rubrics. This refers to imposing categories upon things and seeing things in terms of mental and conceptual categories. In

> **Rubric:** Heading of a part of a book, title, an established rule or custom. A rubric is a frame of reference, a cataloguing that brings and end to an inquiry.

this sense, active attending is a very rare capacity.

What is the problem with dichotomizing? Maslow asserted that "To dichotomize is to pathologize and that within all pathology is dichotomizing." Do this and you distort reality so that you will not see reality as it is. It also creates all sorts of pseudo-problems (self—unselfish, reason —emotion, impulse—control, tragic—comic).

What happens when you stop dichotomizing? You begin to learn to see the wholeness of things—the interconnectedness. By way of contrast, dichotomizing often blinds you to the wholeness of experience. If something doesn't fit into your mental boxes, it doesn't exist—well, for you. When you move beyond the limitations and blindness of dichotomous categories, you often are able to see in such a more holistic and systemic way. You are able to see how one thing relates to another, is a variable within something.

3) Give up Demanding Expectations
Another blinder to pure awareness is expectations. Expectations are often the culprits that undermine and contaminate your ability to purely witness. About this Maslow once commented that "expectations can drown out the voice of reality" (1970, p. 207). When you expect, you impose something on whatever it is that you are experiencing. Yes, expecting is also a resource that enables you to plan and manage your future. It lies at the heart of your ability to predict the possibilities that may occur. So accurate, conscious, and tentative expecting offers you a powerful coping skill.

The problem is not that expectations are bad or wrong in themselves. The problem is that expectations become damaging and problematic when they are textured by demandingness. *Demanding* expectations are those in which you anticipate something *and demand that it occur in a particular way.* Most often, this sets you up for disappointment and disillusionment.

I like the quip of Richard Bandler, "It takes a lot of preparation to feel disappointed." That's because you first have to set up some expectations, then raise the intensity of those expectations by demanding that they have to occur, and then interpret any thing less as terrible, awful, and "the end of your world."

Demandingness is typically coded in words like "must, should, have to" that impose necessities on experiences that are not true requirements. So while I *must* have oxygen, and I *should* get a good night's sleep. Yet in most areas of life my wants and desires turn them into neurotic needs. I may want a raise at work, but to say, "I *must* have that raise." "I *should* be flawless in my spelling." "She *must* get here on time." "He *should* be more thoughtful." Imposing such demands creates unnecessary pressure and blinds you from seeing reality as it is and dealing with it as it is.

4) Freely associate in your thoughts and feelings
So far I have been speaking about witnessing the world, the world of others, and the world that exists outside of you. But if you turn your attention inward, how do you just witness your own experiences? How do you *just observe and witness* what *is* within your own inner world of thoughts, emotions, memories, imaginations, hopes, dreads, etc.?

The problem that now emerges are your mental censors— the higher level beliefs and understandings you hold about what's acceptable and what's not acceptable. It was in the face of censors that Freud invented the technique of free association or thought intrusion. Sigmund Freud invented this technique at the beginning of psychoanalysis. And Maslow (1970, p. 147) spoke about free association as one way to simply witness ourselves.

Free association is meaningful and useful because it allows you to see "the character structure more and more nakedly." (1970, p. 147). If you learn to free associate well, to report without censorship or realistic logic what passes through your consciousness, you will be able to express the structure or form that makes up your character. As Freud designed this, he used the quiet room, the psychoanalytic couch, the permissive atmosphere, and "going with anything that comes to mind," and the releasing of the patient, from all responsibilities as representatives of the culture.

In Neuro-Semantics we often use *the permission frame* to counter the blinding effect of taboo and prohibition frames. By "giving yourself permission" to see, hear, feel, and encounter what you have censored, tabooed, or prohibited, you use a counter-intuitive process. At first it seems like the last thing you would ever want to do. Yet often the problem is the very frame that creates the censoring in the first place.

Permission to be Wrong
If there's any permission that is needed almost universally by human beings, it is the permission to be wrong, to make mistakes, to fail, to mess up. *Wanting* to do things right, in a correct way, to succeed at everything attempted is one thing, *having* to be right about everything is a very different thing. The first is a healthy desire; the second is an unhealthy compulsion that will lock a person up, create rigidity, and generate a pseudo-problem.

I saw this lack of permission very powerfully once during the third module of Meta-Coach, *Coaching Mastery* while in Mexico. It was the last day for the competency-based assessments. Those who had not reached the benchmarked competency of 2.5 on the coaching scale had one more opportunity in a coaching session. I sat in on one coach who was coaching another participant as a client. With the assessment sheet in hand, I was there to do the benchmarking. Now, as you can imagine, in a test situation like this, being watched and being evaluated for your skill competency to determine certification status can generate a lot of performance anxiety. And it did for the young lady I was watching.

Now as a coach, she had already achieved competency of five of the skills and only had two more in which to demonstrate competency. What makes this especially challenging for a coach is that the coach needs to have and experience a purity of presence to a client. And to be totally available for the client, a person has to release all other concerns.

Now the young lady was working with a client who didn't have a clear objective for the session. So as time got away, knowing that the whistle indicating the end of the session would soon be blown, she got more and more agitated.

The client seeing this essentially switched roles and attempted to coach the coach. "What's wrong? Are you okay?" That only made things worse. "I have to reach the benchmark competency level now." she thought. More wasting of the precious moments to demonstrate the needed skills! And then the whistle blew at that very moment. So with all of that there was suddenly an explosion— of tears and statements that she was never going to make it.

Well, obviously to begin the fifteen minutes of debrief was not going to be very productive, she knew she had not succeeded and the feedback would not change that. So I shifted gears to provide support for her as a person. "Are your tears for you not achieving what you wanted to achieve in this session?" I asked. It took a moment, and then out of the tears she said, "No, I'm just so enraged, I'm furious." "And you're enraged about what?"

> "Me!" she said raising her voice. "Me! I'm furious at myself. I just couldn't figure out a way to do the coaching correctly; I'm just so angry at myself."

"Okay, so your rage and anger is directed at yourself for not doing it correctly. Hmmmm. Seems pretty harsh. Do you always treat yourself this way when you don't achieve an important outcome?" Her head was nodding yes as the tears flowed. "And this empowers you as a person!? So what does it mean to you to not do it correctly? Seems like that must be really semantically loaded, like you don't even have permission to do it incorrectly?" And with that the tears really started flowing.

Here she was in the heat of the Crucible— white hot, glowing hot, intense. In fact, we were all there and it only took a few seconds to access it. The trigger that elicited it was the testing experience and the frame that governed the heat that she turned up in those moments was the belief frame that she "*had* to do it right," that she "*had* to do it correctly."

And in the moments we followed, I invited her to try on a permission, *"I give myself permission to do it incorrectly."* She did. And from there some belief frames about mistakes that would allow her to be unconditionally valuable as a human being *and* be a fallible human being who could make mistakes gracefully.

Witnessing to Create Accurate Empathy
What emerges from all of this effort of getting back to pure sensory awareness is a safe and insightful Crucible space. There we can *hold* hot and intense emotions, thoughts, energies, needs, wants, desires, hopes, fears, angers, etc. We can *hold* them because there is no judgment, no evaluation, no meaning-making—just being with the experience as such.

You know you have succeeded in this when you are able to accurately express another person's perspective or emotional state (or your own) to that person's satisfaction. Rogers called this skill "accurate empathy," it is one of the key healing mechanisms that facilitate self-actualization.

In NLP we call this "taking second position." It is one of the *perceptual positions* which describe the various perceptual positions that you can adopt in regard to things. And understanding this position enables you to understand second position.

> *1) First perceptual position.* Typically you look at things from your perspective. You look at things from your eyes, you hear things from out of your ears, you feel things out of your body and skin. *First position* means that you are looking and perceiving and experiencing things from out of yourself. To do this is to know your own thoughts and emotions. It means to have your own voice,

opinion, and perspective. To *only* do this means that you find it hard to understand others and to take their perspective into account.

2) *Second perceptual position* refers to imagining what it would be like to look out of the eyes of another person. It is to "step into his or her shoes and walk a mile." It is to hear, feel, and perceive from the position of the person that you are relating to. When you can do this it gives you the ability to have accurate empathy with that person. To *only* do this is to lose yourself, to not know your own thoughts and emotions, and to always be deferring to others. To not do this is to be locked in to your own perspective and unable to see things from the perspective of others.

3) *Third perceptual position* refers to imagining what you and the other person looks like, sounds like, and feels like from a neutral third party position. It is the "fly on the wall" perspective that we refer to when we say, "I'd like to be a fly on the wall in that meeting." Sometimes this is called the meta-position. To *only* do this is to be stuck in a neutrality state of non-commitment which means that you will be trying to be a "Mr. Spock" (from the Star Trek movies) where you experience little emotion.

4) *Fourth perceptual position* is known as the systems perspective. It is to observe yourself and the other person from the point of view of a system—the organizational system, a cultural system, a historical system, etc. It is sometimes called the "God" or "Universal" perspective. To *only* do this will lead you to become so "up in the air" that you'll be living in LaLa land and less able to apply in everyday life.

From a *second perceptual position* you can more fully understand and describe what a person is thinking, feeling, saying, doing, wanting, etc. It gives you an accurate accounting of the person, one that the person can agree with and when expressed, enables the person to feel heard and understood.

Distinguishing Sensory and Evaluative Data
So how do you learn to witness without judgment? A principle from NLP is that to be *a professional communicator, you have to distinguish sensory based information and evaluative based information.* If you don't do that,

or can't do that, you will make a mess of the communication enterprise. You will contaminate the sensory-based information with your evaluations, and not even realize it.[1] This explains the importance of the Meta-Model, for being able to map out how to distinguish your own inner mappings of things as a meaning-maker from the external facts of the territory that you are mapping. When you do that, then you can ask precision questions that allow you to meet other people at their map of the world, instead of expecting them to meet you at your map.

Sensory data occurs as information and events impact your senses and sense receptors. At first it is outside of conscious awareness. By the time it comes into awareness, you have the "sense" of seeing, hearing, feeling, smelling, and tasting that information. So you can *representationally track* that information to the movie screen of your mind. That's when you begin to make your inner movies—when you bring the world inside your mind and *re-present* it to yourself. This also was the stroke of genius from NLP, that we humans think in the sensory languages of images, sounds, sensations, etc.[2]

Yet all of this is very, very different from *evaluative data*. While both occur in the mind, there is a difference. You first make sensory representations and then you make evaluations about it. This is the meta-stating process of stepping back from yourself, in your mind, and bringing other thoughts and feelings to it. In doing so, you move to a higher level as you draw conclusions, make generalizations, create distortions, make decisions, invent beliefs, and set intentions.

You can tell that you, or another person, has jumped a logical level to the evaluative level if you cannot put what you're talking about with your terms, words, phrases, or language on a table. You can do this if you're using sensory-based words. You put the referents of sensory words on the table, or in a chair, or in a wheelbarrow: chair, dog, green grass, man with large nose. But you cannot put the referents of evaluative language out on the table: "good, bad, brilliant, disappointing, rude, nice, mean, beautiful." As evaluations, these things are creatures of the mind— they only exist in the mind, in the world of communication, not in the outside world.

This is where the questions and distinctions of the Meta-Model provides a tool for creating specificity, precision, and clarity. You use the linguistic distinctions to bring high level evaluations *down* to the representational screen. With the precision questions, you step back down from your matrix of invented reality and back into sensory life.³

This is, however, a challenge. Most of us are easily seduced and hypnotized by evaluative language and do not even know how to make the *sensory/evaluative distinction.* Someone says, "He's mean. He blasted that waiter." And we're off hallucinating and inventing meanings about what those non-specific words means. Out there in the sensory world, there is no "meanness," no "rudeness," no "kindness," no "hurtful," "healing." These are words from the evaluative world of mind. You have to ask such questions as:
- "What do you mean by this word?"
- "How do you know that it is this X?"

Otherwise you will not be "communicating." You will be in a hypnotic trance. Or you will be imposing your trance on others and assuming that the others are creating in their minds the same pictures as you are.

Whenever you accuse someone of being "defensive, hypocritical, incongruent, loving, sensitive, intuitive," or ten-thousand other things, to be masterful at communication you need to immediately *feel* the lack of precision, the inability to track those words directly to the theater of your mind. If you can do that, then you can then begin to explore the other's communication with the precision questions. If you don't, you will be seduced into a story. And to the extent you go into that trance, you are creating more and more mis-understandings and distortions, putting you further and further from clear communication.

Without this *sensory/evaluative* distinction you will simultaneously become a poor communicator and a great mind-reader. You can then even *impose* your judgments on others and never have a clue that you are doing so! With the best of intentions of trying to understand others, you will actually not be seeing them at all, but because you will see them through your filters, you will keep seeing and believing whatever those filters project. Your judgments then come out in subtle ways, in ways that make it almost impossible for the other to push away those impositions.

That's why the kindest and most compassionate thing you can do with your loved ones is to drill in the distinction between *sensory / evaluative data.* When you impose your maps and judgments on others, you are not doing a loving thing.

Taking Second Position to Empathetically Understand
So where are you? Can you intentionally and consciously step out of your own perceptual position (first position) and empathetically stand under (under-stand) another person in supporting him or her? As you step into the other person's perception and take "second position," how well can you imaginatively see and hear things from how they must look like to the person?

When you can simply *witness* what *is*, you can then face reality, deal with the cards dealt you, and make choices with clarity about what to acknowledge, what to change, and what to let go. As a clay crucible doesn't judge or fight with the hot boiling metals poured into it, so you don't judge the intensity of the emotions, needs, or drives. There's no need to. *Such is just the human stuff from which potentials emerge.*

Maslow liked to describe this as the ability to be "a good animal," accepting needs and drives as such, appreciating them for what they offer, and then handling them effectively.

> "See human nature as it is, not as they would prefer it to be. See what is before them without being strained through spectacles of various sorts to distort, shape, or color the reality. Self-actualizing people tend to be good animals, hearty in their appetites, and enjoying themselves without regret or shame or apology. They are able to accept themselves not only on those low levels, but at all levels as well; love, safety, belongingness, honor, self-respect." (*Farther Reaches,* p. 127)

Just *witnessing what is* at the sensory level of experience is not easy. It requires that you "lose your mind" (your meta-mind) and come back to your senses. Strange. You spend your whole life learning to build up distinctions and evaluations so that you can "make sense" of things and then all of that learning then gets in our way from just witnessing what is.

Yet the skill of being able to step out of your meta-mind and return to a pure state of just observing provides you a great resource when that's required. And it is required for this facet of the Crucible.

And when you enter the Crucible, your ability to speak in specific sensory-based language will be your ability to express what you or another is aware of without judgment. For any helper who seeks to facilitate the process, this is critical. While there are times when your judgments and evaluations are important and valuable, it is counter-productive when you are attempting to hold the space for someone. "That's when releasing judgment is required."[4]

Your Crucible Conversation
As you develop your ability to just witness, you will want to build this distinction into your Crucible space. What would best represent "just observing" to you? What other images and/or metaphors convey the idea of "just witnessing" and seeing without judgment? Have you built that into your Crucible?

Crucible Coaching
You won't need your notebook for your first coaching session this week. Instead you'll just need the willingness to play, to be child-again, and to experimental ferociously.

> Imagine that you have been on a journey to another galaxy and you've been away from Earth for two decades. For twenty-years you have talked about the blue sky of earth, the brown and red ground, and the green leaves on trees and plants.
>
> Now you have returned and so go out— look and look, hear and hear, smell and smell, taste and taste, feel and feel. Go out and look at anything and everything *as if for the first time*. Enjoy all of the sensory stimuli that's all around you.

On the surface, just observing what *is* seems like the simplest thing in the world. The reality of actually *just observing and just witnessing* turns out to be one of the most challenging things possible for human beings. The problem is that of *suspending* what you know, what you have experienced, your conclusions, your evaluations, and all of the filters that you have developed. And yet, the ability to "lose your mind and come back to your senses" is an credible resource when it comes to being able to unlearn old things and clear the space for learning new things.

Take time this week to practice just observing. Imagine taking second and third perspective and notice the difference this makes. If you don't have full permission for this, take time to grant yourself this permission. And because the Crucible requires silence and presence, practice being silent as you just observe. Be fully there. Be more fully there then you have ever before.

End of Chapter Notes
1. The Meta-Model is a model of linguistic distinctions and a set of questions to enhance the precision and specificity of a conversation. For a book about that see *Communication Magic* (2001). See the article on www.neurosemantics.com "Being a Professional Communicator."

2. *Movie-Mind* (2001).

3. *Communication Magic* (2001) and *The Structure of Magic, Volumes I and II* (1975, 1976).

4. Releasing Judgment Pattern is in *Sourcebook of Magic, Volume II*.

Chapter 9

ACCEPTANCE

The Magic of Acknowledgment

*"If humanness is accepted and loved,
then many local, ethno-centric problems simply disappear."*
Abraham Maslow (1968, p. 196)

*"Only when his fears are accepted respectfully
can he dare to be bold. We must understand that the dark forces
are as 'normal' as the growth forces."*
Abraham Maslow (1968, p. 54)

"One of the most powerful influences on emotional health and well-being is the capacity to accept reality, to accept what is. The extent to which one can accept what is profoundly affects his psychological ability to adapt."
Joseph Dunn, Ph.D. Psychologist

You do not have to read far in the field of psychology to realize that most psychologists have an amazing appreciation for the awesome power of acceptance. We're always wanting to get people to *accept* themselves, others, life, God, reality, wrinkles, traffic, aging, burnt toast, and other challenges in everyday life.

I learned this surprising secret very early when I came across a quotation from Alfred Alder, and then another from Carl Jung, that I found shocking. Both said, *"You can never get over a neurosis until you can love your neurosis."* My first thought was, "Love your neurosis?" you've got to be kidding! That's the last thing I want to do! "I would never want to encourage anyone to do that!"

While that statement may be an extreme expression designed mostly to shock, it points to an incredibly important resource—*acceptance.* It is, in and through, acceptance that we are healed, released, and freed for emotional health and well-being. The use of the term "love" is used in the first quotation at the top of this chapter to call attention to the absolute necessity of acceptance for solving life's problems. In this, *acceptance,* as a key ingredient for effective coping and for mastering the challenges of life, it is also the pathway to self-actualization. Acceptance surprisingly and paradoxically offers you one of the most powerful transformative tools you'll ever come across. There's hardly anything more profound in human nature than acceptance.

Now if this seems preposterous, recall how acceptance, as a transformative process, has been around a long time and has been known for generations. It is the foundation of serenity prayer:
> "God grant me the serenity to *accept* the things I cannot change, the *courage* to change the things I can, and the *wisdom* to know the difference."

The word *acceptance* (from Latin and French) literally means "to take, receive, or hold." In accepting, you "receive with consent, give admittance, sometimes give approval to, endure without protest, regard as proper, normal, or inevitable, and receive as true." The mental side of acceptance is to receive something into the mind for understanding and comprehension. It is to acknowledge what exists. The emotional side of acceptance involves welcoming something. You don't have to like it, but you do have to welcome it. You have to open the door and invite it in rather than leave it out in the rain.

Abraham Maslow minced no words when it came to his recommendations about acceptance:
> "If we want to be helpers, counselors, teachers, guides, or psychotherapists, what we must do is to *accept the person* and help him learn what kind of person he is already, what is his style, what are his aptitudes, what is he good for, not good for, what can we build upon, what are his good raw materials, his good potentialities?

> We would be *non-threatening* and would supply *an atmosphere of acceptance* of the child's nature which reduces fear, anxiety, and defense to the minimum possible. Above all, we would care for the child, that is, enjoy him and his growth and self-actualization. So far this sounds much like Rogerian therapist, his 'unconditional positive regard,' his congruence, his openness, and his caring." (1970, p. 186, *italics added*)

Maslow also credited acceptance with the power to enable you to more clearly see what's real. For him, acceptance also reduces fear and enables the self-actualizers to live more comfortably with reality as it is. All in all, acceptance enables you to become a friend to reality.

> "The principal reason the self-actualizing person sees reality more clearly is that they see it through an unclouded lens [clean cognizing and meaning-making]. They place no unrealistic, neurotic demands on reality [cognitive distortions]. It is not only the self-actualizing persons see the world as it really is, *they also accept it as it really is.* The result is that they are more comfortable with what they see and less fearful of what they do not see."

> Acceptance enables you to take hold of reality, receive it, and embrace it. It ends the fight that rejection creates.

The Paradox of Acceptance

All of this highlights the paradox of acceptance. *What you accept, you defuse and release.* And conversely, what you do not accept, you fight against and resist. Whatever you resist, you invest with energy. And when you give it the negative energy of resistance, you feed it so that it grows. As the fighting continues it becomes increasingly unmanageable and even overwhelming with the result that it comes to control you. What a nightmare!

The opposite is that of *just accepting* yourself, life, the world, others, the constraints that you face everyday, and the cards life has dealt you. By accepting you invest no negative energy of resistance. You engage in no fight. This is actually the first step to true mastery and empowerment. It is the first step, but not the last.

When you lack acceptance, you lack one of the key ingredients that enables you to face reality. And that undermines your ability to cope with the basic facts of what *is*. When you don't accept something, you go into states of rejecting, denying, repressing, and fighting. You pump your brain full of these kinds of thoughts which puts you at odds with reality. Rather than a friend, you become an enemy to what's real. And the more you continue in this mode, the more you bring non-acceptance thoughts. You do so with unrealistic expectations, impossible desires, and erroneous understandings and all of that will set you up so that as you refuse to face things, you become less and less capable of thinking about them, understanding them, or finding solutions for them. Not a pretty picture. And certainly not the way to unleash your highest potentials.

Acceptance

Pseudo	*Real*
Resignation	Acknowledgment
Low standards	Hold standards while accepting
Tolerance	Neutral welcoming
Abundance and endorsement	Rejection and denial
Abandonment	Welcoming of reality

What is Real Acceptance?
In workshops and in private consultations, I often have a challenge when I try to facilitate participants to see acceptance as a solution. And there's a reason for this. The reason is that over the years, acceptance has gotten a bad rap. How has this come about? It has arisen, in part, due to some of the things that have been associated with, or confused with, acceptance. So to clear the air and restore its reputation, here are a few important distinctions that are essential for fully understanding and fully embracing acceptance. There are several things offered as acceptance which are actually pseudo-acceptance. So what is *real* acceptance?

Acceptance is not resignation. Resignation refers to giving up or giving in. In resignation you lie down and take it. That's not acceptance. In acceptance you welcome into mind and life *with the purpose of effectively responding to it*. In this, acceptance is not complacency or passivity, and it does not indicate the lack of high standards. Again, Dr. Joseph Dunn speaks to this:

> "Acceptance is usually the initial step, and a critical one, in any psychological condition or symptom. Dealing effectively with depression, anxiety, conflict, or destructive habits begins with acceptance. Often the most difficult part of therapy is struggling with resistance to face reality."

Acceptance is not low standards. In accepting you are not lowering your standards, you are acknowledging what *is*. In fact, it is by that acknowledgment of what *is* that you are able to detect the difference between the world as you find it and the high standards that you aim for as you seek to change the world.

Acceptance is not universal tolerance. Acceptance is not just gritting your teeth and tolerating what you despise and/or hate. Paradoxically, it is the lack of acceptance that actually drives perfectionism. Conversely, acceptance of what *is* conquers perfectionism and other forms of mental and emotional intolerance. But this doesn't mean that acceptance is just a form of tolerance. Acceptance more positively *welcomes* facts into awareness, even facts that you might dislike. You welcome in order so that you can more fully understand and take more effective action.

Because in the real world there are all kinds of ambiguities and because there we don't always have neat categories of black-or-white compartments, we are more often able to take effective action when we accept what is.

Acceptance is not endorsement. You can accept something without endorsing it. You can accept a person without approving or endorsing everything that person thinks, feels, or says. Within acceptance is contentment—a contentment with yourself, your lot in life, with the thousands of small pleasures in life. And this basic contentment cuts away intolerance and demandingness.

Acceptance enables you to welcome life circumstances all the while taking proactive steps to create the life you want. So in releasing what you cannot control, you are then able to focus more fully on what you want. So another paradox: Acceptance facilitates in you a more proactive stance and responsible stance in life.

Acceptance is not abandonment. In acceptance you let another person *be* him or herself and responsible. No wonder acceptance is critical for relationships because without it, people are trying to change each other. And that creates several problems, not the least of which is allowing each person to take responsibility for their own change. Conversely, acceptance enables you to suspend your defenses and judgments that interfere with accurate perceptions. Relationally, the ability to live with differences depends upon your ability to accept and the quality of that acceptance.

The Power of Acceptance
Acceptance facilitates forgiveness. In fact, you can think of forgiveness as an acceptance grace. By forgiving, you are able to come to terms with major hurts that you cannot just dismiss as if they are nothing. When you accept that another has violated something important and you have addressed it so that it won't be repeated, your acceptance acknowledges what happened and releases it. So it does not contaminate you or your spirit. You accept that the other messed up, violated an important value to you, *and* you also accept that it is done and over. Now you can let it go. That's forgiveness. You do not hold the event in your mind or memory against someone or even against yourself.

Acceptance facilitates humor. Acceptance also lies at the heart of healthy humor and laugher, it enables you to lighten up and laugh at yourself. Humorist Woody Allen illustrates a humorous acceptance, "I wasn't born a good looking kid, I didn't acquire these looks until later in life." This humor at himself, at his looks, both allows him to more fully accept himself and expresses that acceptance. Acceptance is required if you want to lighten up, laugh things off, and not take yourself so seriously.

Acceptance facilitates humanness. In these ways acceptance enables you to treat people as real live human beings. When you stop confusing what people *do* with who they *are* as human beings, you transcend the need to judge them. Judgment is one of those "horses of the apocalypse" for relationships according to research John Gottman. It absolutely prevents the creation of the safe space in the Crucible. People need a real or authentic space where they can allow what *is* to just be—without judgment. When you accept people as real live human beings, fully fallible, you can then support them by *just witnessing* their reality of what is as you support them dealing with it and moving to transformational change and solution.

Accessing a Robust State of Acceptance
- What challenges you in terms of accepting?
- What problems or situations do you find yourself fighting against intolerance of which you know you can't change?
- About what do you say "I can't stand...?"
- How well do you accept yourself with all of your imperfections and fallibilities?
- How well do you accept your world or others?

If acceptance is such a powerful and healing influence as a state and as a frame of mind, how do you learn to fully access it? How do you practice it? Is it a robust experience for you? How can you develop more ready access to it and use it when you need it?

1) Identify something small and simple to accept. The art of accessing acceptance starts in the mind as a way of thinking and perceiving. Begin by noticing what you already accept that you could just as easily reject. Think of something small and simple that you accept. How about the rain, traffic in a big city, lines at the airport, the baby's diaper needing to be changed, taking out the garbage? Or you can think about something that you once did *not* accept, but rejected, hated, and found intolerable and then over the years, you gave up the fight and now just simply accept it.

2) Experience that event fully in your body. As you think about something small that you accept, see and hear it on the theater of your mind until you are able to step into that experience and feel it in your body. When you do, notice how you are breathing, your muscle tension, your gestures, movements, voice, tone, eyes, face, etc. Take a snapshot of what this experience of acceptance feels like and how you know it somatically. To learn this even better, think of something that you definitely do not accept. Do the same with it, see and hear it until you step in and feel it, then take a snapshot of that state. Are these different states?

3) Adopt the language of acceptance. As you experience acceptance, notice the language of acceptance and as you do, contrast that to the language of non-acceptance (i.e., rejection). When you don't accept you typically utilize the language of *can't*.

> "I can't stand to fail, that would be terrible." "I can't stand to be laughed at." "I can't tolerate having to wait."

These are *psychological can'ts,* not actual limitations and constraints, as in "I can't fly." *Psychological can'ts* drive your intolerance and non-acceptance and indicate frames of prohibition which taboo the experience that you are considering. To undo the damage of prohibition, there's a radical operation needed: you need to step up and *give yourself permission.*

> "I give myself permission to fail." "I give myself permission to be human, fallible, to live in a fallible world, to make mistakes, to learn from them, to make the most of things," etc.

I had to learn this when my dad died. When I got the message, I went for a run to think about things and as I did, I could hear a soft inner voice saying, "I can't believe it." True, words of his death came as a shock; it was surprising and unexpected. And sure, it was not something I was ready for. But the truth I needed to tell myself was, "I could and would believe it." True enough, I didn't want to. But I did. I welcomed the fact of his death because I didn't want to make myself an enemy to reality. If it's real, I'll befriend it.

4) Re-set your frames from the intolerance to acceptance. Re-setting your frames from the intolerance, perfectionism, and taboos via giving yourself permission opens you up to acceptance. Simply continue to do so until it becomes a felt reality within you, until it becomes emotional acceptance. This is the power of changing your internal dialogue. Dr. Joseph Dunn writes:

> "Real acceptance involves being open to emotionally absorb or digest *what is.* There is an absence of emotional defensiveness and avoidance."

Dr. Dunn is not the only person to use the metaphor of digestion. Fritz Perls used it extensively in his development of Gestalt therapy. In fact, he listed as one of the defense mechanism—introjection. *Introjection* refers to taking an experience in whole without digesting it. Perhaps it was so overwhelming, so confusing, or perhaps it occurred too quickly to be processed. But whatever the cause, a person introjects an experience as a whole without reflection and full understanding to decide what to accept of it and what to reject. Like trying to swallow food whole without chewing it up, without breaking it up so that it can be digested, an introjected experience lies inside— unused, undigested, and therefore stuck.

The bottom line about acceptance is that acceptance is a mental and emotional state. While there are spiritual traditions that have rituals that take years to achieve in terms of achieving acceptance, it doesn't have to be that difficult. Nor does the "stages of grief resolution" have to be so long and hard. In Elizabeth Kubler-Ross analysis of the grief stages, a person moves from shock, denial, bargaining, depression, and finally moves on to (guess what? Yes!) acceptance. Yet if acceptance is just a mind-body state, why not just start there with it as a resource?

Every mind-body-emotion state is simply that——a *state* of mind, of body, and emotion. And when you know that, you have two "royal roads to state" —mind, body.[1] You have what you're thinking and how you're using your physiology. That's why "thinking about a time when . . ." you had an experience of acceptance with something small and simple and noticing the state of your body in all of its dimensions empowers you to access *acceptance* and use it to set *accepting frames of mind* about other things.

My Divorce Crucible
The life experience that served as a terrible crucible for me, one I did not choose, one for which I was not ready, occurred early in my life and entailed the shock and devastation of divorce. I was young when it happened, 25, but I felt old. I felt as if it was "the end of life as I knew it." Surprisingly, that wasn't far from the truth.

And because I refused to accept the divorce and because I fought it with everything within me, I did not learn from it or use the experience as productively as I could have. I fought it because I thought by fighting for the marriage and against the divorce, that would restore things. It didn't work out that way.

So the negative experience stayed inside me as an unacceptable part —an experience I didn't come to terms with and that I would not let be. Much of what kept me from accepting and learning from it were my own taboos about divorce. After all, at the time I was a young minister. "How could that happen to me?" How could God allow that to happen to me?" My questioning itself encoded the language of non-acceptance which, in turn, locked me into fighting and resisting instead of accepting reality as it was.

Obviously as long as I was asking those kinds of questions, I wasn't accepting responsibility and without responsibility I was not learning what I needed to learn. Slowly I did take responsibility for my part and so I did learn— a bit. I learned what I could learn at the time, but there were more learnings to come!

Why? Because at one level I was still fighting it. It took the second marriage and divorce to come fully to accept it and to see my contributions as well as the cultural frames that contributed and which also set me up for the not accepting that sometimes people grow apart. I would have taken my non-accepting attitude into the Crucible and worked it through so that life wouldn't have had to serve that purpose.

Accessing Acceptance

1) Identify an experience of acceptance.
>When have you just accepted something for what it *is*?
>What do you now accept that once you fought, rejected, and hated?
>How does your current acceptance improve the quality of your life?

2) Fully access the experience.
>What do you see, hear, and feel when you recall that accepting experience?
>How much do you feel the state of acceptance?
>What would make it stronger for you?
>What is it like in your body? Breathing, gestures, movements, etc.?

3) Set an anchor for this state.
>Link some special word, gesture, symbol, etc. for this state.
>Step in and out of the state until you can trigger the anchor and quickly get back into state.

4) Apply the acceptance to another area where you need and want acceptance.
>What other area of life are you non-accepting, judgmental, intolerant, rejecting, resigning?
>Trigger the anchor of your acceptance state and hold as you link that state with whatever you want to be more accepting.

Learnings about Acceptance

There's hardly another state as healing or freeing as acceptance. It powerfully enables you to adjust yourself to reality for what it *is* which then enables you to take the next step in moving forward with a positively creative response.

Ultimately, *acceptance* is a state and because it is, you can use the tools and processes of state accessing and applying to access the state and use it to set new *frames of mind* about other areas of life where acceptance would free and renew you.

Your Crucible Conversation
To bring acceptance into your conversation with yourself and others, what language expressions will you adopt that will best express this for you? How thoroughly do you distinguish acceptance from condoning or resigning? What images and metaphors do you want to use for acceptance? A menu list of possibilities: a mailbox, open hands, shrugging of the shoulders, big sign that says, "OK!"

Crucible Coaching
Okay, coaching time again. Now with your notebook, *My Transformational Life,* devote a page to "Things I Can't Change."

> If you can't change what you won't accept, make a list of things that you need to just accept? Make a list of all the factors outside your control and influence. How well have you now made crystal clear distinctions in your mind about acceptance and distinguished it from resignation, tolerance, endorsement, and abandonment?
>
> Take time this week to practice accessing a pure and simple state of acceptance. Record the number of times throughout each day that you just accepted something and moved on to do what you could about the situation. Record the times when you got upset and frustrated and perhaps in a strong dislike, even hate, and rejection when you could have saved yourself all of that trouble if you had just accepted what *is* and then looked around for some way to cope with it.

End of Chapter Notes:
1. This is a basic NLP distinction that you can find in any introduction book to NLP: *Sourcebook of Magic, Movie Mind, User's Manual for the Brain, Volume I.*

Chapter 10

TRUTH

The Heart of Authenticity

*"The first act of courage is simply to see things as they are.
No excuses, no explanations, no illusions of wishful progress."*
Peter Block

"You shall know the truth and the truth will set you free."
Jesus Christ, Gospel of John

"To be completely honest with oneself is the very best effort
a human being can make."
Sigmund Freud

Truth is the central element of the Crucible. It is central because it is the element that generates the heat and the fire within the Crucible. You don't have to add any heat, truth is enough to heat things up! That's because truth, as that which is real, genuine, and authentic, cleanses us from everything false and so makes us genuinely alive. Truth increases our aliveness enabling us to become *real* persons.

Will Schutz, a leader in the HPM, described the power of truth-telling in the Crucible encounter in terms of a metaphor with some very vivid language:
"Telling the truth pops the cork. Out flows the person. Lying blocks self-insight and interpersonal contact. Lying blocks exploration of the self." (*Profound Simplicity*, p. 69)

In terms of self-actualizing, Maslow urged, "When in doubt, be honest." And Fritz Perls went further when he wrote:

> "A little bit of honesty goes a long way and this is what most of us are afraid of — being honest with ourselves and stopping the idea of self-deception." (*Witness to Therapy,* p. 127)

It is here that we develop the courage to speak the truth, to be ruthlessly honest, and to not only see and recognize what's real, but speak and live what is real. And it is the action of *speaking* and *living* truth that increases the very energy that can become heat within the Crucible. Why? Because these actions of speaking and living truth can be scary— they can be dangerous to life as we know it.

The truth here is not Truth with a capital T. It is not absolute or ultimate truth. It is not God's truth. It is *your* truth; it is *my* truth. It is the truth or reality of our lives, our emotions, our struggles, our perceptions and of this moment. Truth is the inner sense of rightness, of coherence, of completion, of doing what's right, fair, and just.

The Crucible Question
"Is that Your Truth?"
The question to ask when you get inside the Crucible is a simple one, and yet one that many people find challenging to ask, *"Is that your truth?"* But the key will be to ask it repeatedly. In fact, it is the iteration of this question, time after time, level upon level, that enables and empowers this question so that in the Crucible, you discover the truths hidden deep within your cognitive unconscious.[1]

The man before me, Bill, came to the Self-Actualization Workshop of *Unleashing Potentials* and his opening choice on day one for unleashing was to be unleashed *from* some fears of launching his new business and unleashed *to* financial success. By the second day, he had explored his matrix of meaning and reordered several meanings that gave him a greater sense of freedom and control. But there was something else going on within him.

"So what would you like to take into the Crucible? What needs to be melted down and reformulated? Or what experience has not been fully integrated and somehow holds you back?" He said it was his anger at his dad. "Okay, so would you like to take your anger at your dad into the Crucible?" He said he would.

I asked him about his Crucible. "Where is your Crucible?" It was a special room in an ideal house that he had been imagining. I then asked what it looked like and how he had put the concentric circles of safety and encounter into it.

"Okay, so are you ready?" He said he was. "Then let's bring 'anger at dad' into this Crucible . . . and as you do, knowing deep within yourself that your anger is just that, an emotion about something and that you are so much more than your emotions and your anger. And as you bring this 'anger at dad' in, what happens when you *just witness* it without judgment, just curious and interested in one or more events of your anger, and as you now *just acknowledge and accept* that you have had anger at your dad, what are you now aware of?"

> "[Hesitating and coughing] . . . Ah, just that I'm angry ... very angry. He should never have done what he did!!"

"And Bill, let me remind you of your witnessing place in your house, that place in front where you can look down upon the estate and just see it, and as you go there now— feel that pure witnessing ... that's right... [nodding] ... you got it? [nodding yes] ... good, and being in that place, now witness that anger and its object, and now what are you aware of?"

> [Quietly] "That I have been carrying this for a long time."

"So is that your truth Bill—that he should not have done those things and this is the source of your anger that you've been carrying this for a long time?"

> "Yes, he was wrong and should have been stopped."

"Oh, so that's your truth, 'He was wrong; he should have been stopped!'? And if that's your truth, and what else are you aware of?"

> "That little children are innocent and should be treated with respect and care."

"Hmmmm, so is that your truth— 'Little children are innocent and should be treated with respect and care!'?" . . . Hmmmm and now what are you aware of?"

> "[Crying and sobbing] . . . it was so unfair. I didn't have a chance with that. It's held me back . . ."

"And as you just witness and just acknowledge that he should never have done what he did, and that you're very angry at him for what he did . . . just noticing that, what else are you aware of?"

> "That he really *should not have done the things he did.*"

"And now that you have said that out loud— 'He should not have done what he did,' [I repeated raising my voice and using a tone of voice similar to how Bill said it] and as you are with that awareness now—an awareness that you've been carrying a long time— just acknowledging it with acceptance, now what are you aware of Bill?"

> "That I have been sabotaging myself because of this; thinking that I was the one who was wrong and bad."

"Is that your truth? Is this your reality and is this what is truly authentic with you?"

> "Well. . . No. . . The truth is that *I took that experience and interpreted it* in a way so that I made myself bad, I made myself wrong. I've been the one buying the B.S.! I've been the one thinking that I was dirty and unclean. But I wasn't, it was his stupidity!" [Now raising his voice almost to the point of yelling.]

"So is that your truth? Is your truth that you have mis-interpreted things and created a self-image of being bad, dirty, wrong, unclean? Is that your truth?"

> "Yes, that's my truth."

"Great! What can you appreciate in that? What was the positive intention that drove you to do what you now realize was self-sabotage—a mistake?"

> "Appreciate? Nothing. He should not have done that! I should kill him for what he did! I should make him pay for what he did!"

"So accepting this level of anger, it is anger— hot and intense anger, justifiable anger, what now is your truth?"

> [Pause] ". . . yes . . . no . . . he was just acting out of his own pain... he was..."

[I pause while Bill took half a minute to process his thoughts and emotions. As he did I quietly repeated the places in his ideal house where he encoded the resource states of his Crucible.] "So is that your truth, that he was just acting out of his own pain? [A whispered "Yes."] So what will you do about that?"

> [Shouting] "It's over! It's done and over with! . . . [crying and wiping away tears] I'm free; I don't have to be living my life in the shadow of my dad or his craziness, his anger, his stupidity. That's his stuff!"

"So is that your truth?"
"Yes! Definitely! That's my truth."

"And. . . ?"
"Well, I'm free to launch my business and get on with things and succeed! Back then I was doing the best I could at that time; it was just a mistake—a big one, but a mistake. I was just a kid when I created those beliefs, so what do you expect? I now realize that it was those stupid beliefs that was the real problem."

"So that's your truth—that you've mis-interpreted things, created stupid beliefs, and you can now value and appreciate your heart, your intentions, and that now—today—you are free to get going with your business! That your anger at your dad's dysfunction has nothing to do with you and your life today?!"
"Yes."

"So what will you do? What will this truth, this realization, this appreciation enable you now to do to more fully do than you've been able to do before now?"
"I'll launch my business as I've been mapping it out here and give it my all. Nothing to stop me now!"

"You sound excited. Is this your passion, what is true for you at this time?"
"Absolutely!"

"So what are you ready to fall in love with or what have you fallen in love with?"
"Well, my business *and my life* . . . especially my life. . . . This is great! Thank you so much!"

"It's been my pleasure. So thank you, and . . . welcome to the land of the unleashed!" [Applause]

The Velveteen Rabbit

Late at night in a child's bedroom, a Skin Horse and a stuffed Rabbit sit up and talk about what it means to be real.

The Skin Horse says, "Real isn't how you are made; it's a thing that happens to you. When a child loves you for a long, long time, not just to play with but really loves you, then you become real."

"Does it hurt?" asks the Rabbit.

"Sometimes," says the Skin Horse, for he was always truthful. "When you are real, you don't mind being hurt."

"Does it happen all at once, like being wound up, or bit by bit?"

"It doesn't happen all at once," said the Skin Horse. "You become. It takes a long time. That's why it doesn't often happen to people who break easily, or who have to be carefully kept. Generally, by the time you are real, most of your hair has been loved off, and your eyes drop out and you get loose in the joints and very shabby. But these things don't matter at all, because once you are real, you can't be ugly, except to the people who don't understand."

Margery Williams
The Velveteen Rabbit

The Iteration of the Truth Question

What is true? What is real? Because we can be blinded and deceived in so many ways, we can easily lose our way and not know the truth— not know our own truths. Isn't that incredible? That's the reason for repeatedly asking the truth question again and again. And it is in repeating time after time the truth question, "Is that your truth?" that you are able to move a person beyond the first level, the shallow truths, and up the levels of truth with the deeper truth. This *process question* provides you a significant way to get to the real truth or at least be high enough level of truth that will make a transformative difference.

> "Truth occurs in our engagement with the world. ... true understanding is the result of human engagement, for there is no 'pure truth' that lies outside human engagement with the world ... we know through interaction and engagement."
>
> Donald Polkinghorne
> on Heidegger's view

In the example with Bill, his first truth was at too low a level to be helpful. It may have been true that his dad was wrong and abusive, but so what? This "truth" is a complaint about someone else. So while he had his truth, it was driven by rejection (not acceptance), personalizing (not witnessing), hatred (not appreciation), and blame (not responsibility). So I danced with him to facilitate him using these new resources and rising up to higher level truths.

The goal in the Crucible is to get to the "real truth"—the deeper truth —and to find the heart of the matter for yourself or for others. *The heart of the matter for you will be the meanings that you have adopted or created.* It will be the meanings that now define your life, govern your reality, and set the frames for your responses. Yet getting to those meanings, the real beliefs and meanings and understandings, the cognitive unconscious within you, is seldom an easy task. Defenses stand in the way; deceptions block the path to the light and your ability to jump to the next reflective level.

> His first truth was at too low a level to be helpful.

Defenses to Save You from the Truth

Traditional psychology came up against the ego-defenses early in its development. Then Freud and others began mapping out all of the ways that we defend ourselves against ourselves. Ultimately they mapped out a whole set of *defense mechanisms* to explain how we protect and defend ourselves from really knowing ourselves and being honest, truthful, and genuine with ourselves.

And why do we do that? We defend ourselves precisely because when we don't feel safe or capable, we lack the ego-strength (a strong sense of self) to be able to face the threatening nature of reality. To know the truth makes demands on us, asks that we change, grow, and own up to the facts. So we defend ourselves. We protect ourselves by using such defense mechanisms as—

- Rationalization and intellectualization.
- Denial and refusal to consider things (stubbornness).
- Projection of our fears and worries onto others.
- Introjection of something "whole" without digesting it.
- Desacralization as we discount precious things (love, joy, hope, tenderness, small steps).

Now this primarily applies for people who are not psychologically whole or mature, who do not have a robust sense of self so that they can face unpleasant truths. Yet to a lesser degree, it applies to all of us—even to the psychologically healthy. We also defend ourselves and we all also have blind spots. No one is without blind spots. Every strength creates them, every weakness, every meta-program, every model, and every belief. We also lack full self-awareness and often distrust our capacities for handling the challenges of life.

> "How much of your dignity and pride depend on concealment and secrecy? How would you feel if people could always read your mind and know what you were thinking all the time? Or, if they could physically see you at all times— naked, without privacy or concealment, in all your private and secret activities? The dignity and pride that would then remain are your only *real* dignity and pride."
> Abraham Maslow
> (1996: p. 75)

As a result, when you begin speaking your truths, you speak *first level truths* —easy truths, gentle truths, obvious truths, surface truths, truths that blame others and circumstances. You speak truths you can handle, that you can cope with. It is for this reason that we iterate the truth question as we hold the space. This enables the person in the fierce conversation to move up to higher and higher levels of truth (or deeper and deeper truths if you prefer that metaphor).

There's a reason behind this madness. *Truth comes in levels.* It begins with the surface truths that you speak, the truths of your conscious mind, the obvious facts, insights, beliefs, and understandings that you are quick to identify. Then there are the truths in the back of your mind *about* your first level truths. These are the truths that support, enable, and govern your first level truth. These are the presuppositions and assumptions behind and above those truths. So getting to these higher level truths enable you to move up the levels of your mind and find the "belief system," or the matrix of meanings that you live in and operate from.[2]

You can then move up the levels through the iteration of the simple questions: "Is that your truth?" "And what are you know aware of?" "And what comes to mind when you focus on that?" As we do this, we open up the matrix of truths embedded in the lower level truths. This enables you and anyone you work with to move up beyond what you're conscious about to what's in your beyond-conscious-mind.

And as you spiral upward to the truths that have been guiding and informing your lives, you get to the heart of the matter. And the heart of the matter are those governing meanings, usually outside-of-conscious awareness ("unconscious") that are your personal premises and assumptions about yourself, others, and life.

In terms of adult learning, this process enables you to step back repeatedly and draw a next-level conclusion from your previous conclusions. It enables you to take an experience and reflect upon it time and again so that you can harvest many learnings from it and then choose the learnings that best support you and your development.

Getting to the Source
The question I'm always asked at this point is, "And how do you know when you get to the source?" And before I can answer, another one follows quick on its heels: "How can I know that I'm not just fooling myself and deceiving myself thinking it is the highest truth when it is not?"

There's a couple of answers to this. The first is that, at one level, it doesn't matter. What is important is that you take whatever level of truth that you find, and take it to the next resources of appreciation and responsibility. "What do you appreciate about this? What are you going to do now?" Doing this enables you to test the "truth" and work with that level of truth and that allows the person's values (appreciation) and responsive actions (responsibility) to emerge.

Even if the truth is not your highest truth, or the ultimate truth, it is a level of truth—perhaps the most truth you can say to yourself at that moment. It is probably a higher level truth than what you have been aware of, and by being with it and making it conscious, you give yourself a chance to discover what you can do with it. And even if it is not a higher level of truth, you are at least speaking your truth out-loud, and that's a healthy step. It gives you a chance to hear it! Later you can revisit the Crucible and iterate the truth question again and see where it then takes you. So there's no need to worry if you don't resolve everything in one session.[3]

Further, if the truth is not a higher insight that opens up new possibilities, then the appreciation and responsibility questions that follow will reveal that. They will send you back to another iteration of the truth question. In this way the process continues to open you up increasingly to yourself. It will open up at a rate and speed just right for you. So relax, sit back, and just go with the experience.

And what about the concern regarding self-deception? That too will open up more and more as the process continues, as you bring acceptance and explanation to yourself. Now the biggest sign that you have gotten to the top and found a new revolutionary truth for yourself is the emergence of a great insight or a peak experience. Suddenly you have a breakthrough! Suddenly you gain an awareness that opens up a whole new life, a whole new way of responding, love, joy, ecstasy, humor, lightness, transcendence, etc. When that happens, the truth that you found is setting you free and pointing to the door, that will next facilitate your unleashing.

Truth and Authenticity
Finding your truth is searching for, identifying, and then living what is real and authentic for you. It is this that enables *you* to be authentic. And it is *being* real in yourself that enables you to find the life and the way of responding that enables you to be true to yourself. And, of course, that's a description of integrity and honesty.

And in this context, I'm speaking about *being real to your highest self,* not your lowest. If you don't keep asking the questions, you can stop at a lowest self "truths" which actually can create bondage and limitations. "I must be true to my emotions" is one of the lowest self truth on the same order of "I must be true to all of my impulses, needs, drives, and thoughts."

At best that can only lead to a "cave man authenticity." It is the "authenticity" of wanting sex with someone and acting on it regardless of whether the other wants it or its consequences. It is the "authenticity" of wanting to hit, hurt, or kill another because you're upset, angry, or humiliated. You feel it, you want to do it, and you are "real" when you act on your basest instincts *and* you are only living at the animal level, not the human level of self-actualization. And yet it is often a level of truth that you must first go through in order to go higher.

I put "authenticity" in quotes in the previous paragraph because it is a not being authentic to your inner self or highest self (your real self), just some temporary and undeveloped impulse. It is being real to your lowest self, your animal self. At a higher level to the primary thoughts, emotions, impulses, drives, and needs that pop into your awareness are your highest values, visions, principles, and ethics. It is the *being*-values of the self-actualization level that makes you most real, most authentic, most yourself. And that is the true self that you are seeking to unleash, nurture, and develop.

Facing the Truth
When Rocky Balboa (of the Rocky movies, played by Sylvester Stallone) lost to Clubber Lang and his manager Micky dies, Apollo Creed became Rocky's new manager. But Rocky no longer had the "eye of the tiger." That's what Apollo said to him, "You have lost your edge." So to get his edge back, Rocky agreed to go back to basics and learn from Apollo. But it did not seem to be working. Something was wrong.

Then one day while running on the beach and feeling defeated, Andrea confronted Rocky. "Tell me the truth" she said. "Why did you come here?"
 "It's over." Rocky mumbled, almost under his breath.
"You've never quit anything since I have known you."
 "It's so bad."
"What's so bad?" she said raising her voice pleadingly.
 "Micky died ... the fights were rigged. Just hang on to the title."
"He loved you — protected you."
 "I'm just a loser."
"It was real!" she affirmed, again raising her voice.
 "I didn't believe in myself."
"Why don't you tell me the truth?"
 "I don't care ... I didn't want to lose."
"What's the truth, damn it?" she demanded.
 "I'm afraid. For the first time in my life."
"Nothing wrong with fear."
 "It is for me."

"Yet was real. That's a lie. Get rid of it. You're alive. Look at what it's doing to you now. You have to want to do it— for yourself."

"If I lose?"

"You lose ... without fear, without excuses.

"How did you get so tough?"

"I live with a fighter!"

The Fierce Conversation

When you find the truth, then what? What do you do with truth is *speak it*. By first speaking truth first to yourself, you let that truth effect you. You live it. You act on it. And I won't trick you—speaking the truth to yourself is a tough challenge. Actually, it is one of the ultimate challenges that any of us ever experience. That's also why speaking the truth in the safe space of the Crucible facilitates a fierce conversation that gets to the heart of things. And this is part of what creates the intensity of the heat that you experience in the Crucible. Why? Because this entails the courage to face yourself fully and completely and when you do that you are inviting change.

Speaking truth out loud taps into the power of defusing. That is, you can often release things that you have not yet accepted by simply saying out loud what's been eating at you on the inside. Aristotle said, "That which is expressed is impressed." Saying it out loud can help to relieve inner tensions. That's why all of us at times yell and cry and say stupid things and after we get it out of our system we feel better and what we said we recognize as just "being stupid" and meant nothing. We were just unloading and defusing ourselves.[4]

I mentioned earlier that Carl Rogers missed something. Now is the time to say what I think he missed. He missed one of the most important and critical facets of a Crucible. *He missed* **what to do** *with the safety, warmth, empathetic understanding space that he discovered.* He missed *using* that space for engaging in a direct conversation that gets to the heart of the client's difficulties or responsibility for unleashing potentials. He missed speaking the truth about what's real and directing the unleashing process. Presupposing that change would just organically occur, he failed to see the importance of *guiding a fierce conversation about a person's meanings*. He missed it because he assumed that the person would just naturally self-actualize, naturally embrace the truth, and that there would be no need for guidance.

While that is sometimes true, there are also times we need directions. Sometimes we need guidance about what to do and how to do it.

Sometimes we really do not know—don't have the knowledge, have not made the critical distinctions, and/or don't know the pathway for our next step. This is especially true regarding our fullest development and self-actualization. Without instincts, we don't know how to become fully human/ fully alive. That's why we need mentors and coaches to guide us along the way.

Confronting Two or More Truths
Sometimes you will experience two truths—two frames, meanings, beliefs, decisions, interpretations, etc., two that are contradictory in the same time-space moment. What then? What do you do when you have an old truth that you "know" is true at the emotional and body level but intellectually you know is not true? What do you do when, intellectually, you know the opposite is actually true?

While this may sound like a rare experience, it is actually a very common one. It is one that we all frequently experience. As you learn something new and different, you seek to update your maps of reality and yet sometimes the new doesn't go in, it doesn't click in fully? Why not? Because some old "truth" is blocking it.

At such times, the solution is to facilitate a *truth confrontation*. There's several ways to do this. The first and most obvious way is simply to question and challenge the old truth that doesn't serve you well:
    Is this true? Really?
    Do you absolutely know that it is true? That it is always true?
    If it were absolutely true, what would that mean to you?
    What evidence do you have that it is not true?
    Is it true or is it just something that you are familiar with?

Another way to facilitate a truth confrontation is to intentionally invite yourself (or another) to face the two contradictory truths at the same time. The design will be to facilitate *cognitive dissonance*. This is what you feel when there's an internal conflict and incongruence between two ideas, two feelings, two choices. And because none of us like the tension of the incongruence, there's a natural tendency to reduce the cognitive dissonance by changing one or the other of the ideas, feelings, or choices.[5]

Here you'll use cognitive dissonance to disconfirm the old felt-truth by a new truth that you want to commission to govern your mind-body system. The process will be to get in touch with both truths and, as you do, to feel each vividly and fully. As you are with each, welcome each to become visceral and embodied. Then juxtapose the two. And when you do, they will jar and conflict! Let them. Let the tension of the conflict and incongruency arise. Paradoxically, and probably surprisingly, it will depotentate the old felt truth that you don't want to be running your system. To facilitate this, state the old truth out loud. Do it repeatedly. State it as a command.

Meaningfulness
Self-actualization is a function of synthesizing rich and robust meanings with effective performances. That was the discovery that I made about self-actualization and wrote about in my first book on the *subject—Unleashed!* (2007). If self-actualization is about meaning, about rich and robust meanings, then *what sets you free is finding the truth*. Freedom comes from having a fiercely honest conversation that gets to the heart of meaning. When that happens, you then discover the driving influences within you and the leverage points for change. Of course, to do that requires that you cut through the roles, personas, excuses, "reasons," "explanations," justifications, and defenses. This is where speaking your truth and facilitating the emergence of another's truth comes in.
• What does it mean to "get to the heart of things?"
• What does it mean to have a fierce conversation that's transformational enough to unleash potentials?
• How is it that you can get a conversation to open up and reveal the meta-leverage points for change?

If what lies at the heart of all things human is *meaning,* and if meaning is *not* given in our nature, then none of us innately know what anything means. This is our greatest dilemma— and our most precious opportunity. To discover what anything means, we have to learn. We have to explore. We have to ask, reason, interview, invent, and imagine. We have to have a conversation with ourselves that gets to the heart of the meanings that we have inherited, absorbed unconsciously, and that we have consciously created. Only then can we truly talk about the meanings that we want to create and live. This is what the fierce conversation is all about.

To facilitate this in Neuro-Semantics, we begin with the NLP and Meta-States Communication Models and these allow us to get to the heart of things in the conversation of precision. *The Crucible* facilitates the transformational "dialogue" so that meaning (*logos*) will move through (*dia*) us as we communicate to expose the heart of the matter. Failure to do this, and there will be no true dialogue, only talk. Only monologues— preaching the problem! The conversation will go nowhere. The conversation will not be a coaching conversation that gets to the heart of the matter.

Doing this also makes a conversation fierce. The conversation becomes fierce in focus. *That's because the heart of the matter is what matters to you.* The conversation puts you in touch with your inner essence, with your uniqueness, with your particular vision and values, and as such creates a moment of existential awareness. It gets to the heart of the *meanings* that you have absorbed or created for yourself or that you want to create.

When you have done that, you can then powerfully *quality control* your meanings. You can check the quality of the meaning and how well it fits your life—how well it empowers and enhances. The reason for this is that there are levels of meaning and low level meaning creates a low level life.[6]

Again, what enables this conversation is the safety of knowing that you are more than your behaviors, that your worth and dignity and value is unconditionally given, and you can be open and vulnerable to the eyes of another. Here you can be ruthlessly compassionate and speak the truth to *facilitate the unleashing of hidden potentials*.

Are you Ready for this?
Jack Nicolas played a Colonel opposite of Tom Cruise in the movie, "A Few Good Men." The dramatic turning point in the courtroom came when Cruise, a young military lawyer, said he just wanted the truth. Nicolas responded angrily, "You want the truth? You can't handle the truth!"

> The truth will set you free, but first it will make you sweat and will annoy the hell out of you!

How about you? Can you handle the truth of your life and your meanings? Yes, the truth will set you free, but first it will make you sweat! You may even sweat blood and tears before you fully own up to your truths. Most of us do it that way. As crazy as it is—we fight the very truths that will free us and empower us!

It's been said that while "the truth will set you free," it will first annoy the hell out of you! Why? Probably because there are some truths that you don't want to be true, you wish they are not the truth. And also, the thing about truth, as with light, it exposes. Truth turns on the light so that you see what previously you could easily avoid by keeping it in the darkness.

We fight it like Jacob wrestled with the angel.[7] Jacob was caught by surprised one night when the angel of the Lord attacked him. And as they fought, the angel put Jacob's hip out of place. He wounded him. So Jacob grabbed the angel; he clutched him and refused to let him go until he gave him a blessing. This dynamic happens with you also. When you wrestle with truth, you will often feel wounded, exposed, put out of joint, changed, handicapped. But if you persist, if you don't let it go, the truth will bless you.

Wrestling with truth is worth it. In the end, you'll not only be free, you'll be powerful, you'll be genuine, and you'll be your best self. Truth is not your enemy. After all, what is real, actual, and true will ultimately be found out. So the sooner you face reality as it is, the sooner you can get on with your life and your self-actualization.

Crucible Coaching
In your notebook, devote a page to "Defenses Against the Truth." Now make a list of your typical defenses, the way that you seek to escape from the truth.

> How do you usually defend yourself from facing truths that are unpleasant or undesirable? How clear are you that these defenses or escapes do not serve you well in the long-term? How willing are you to commit yourself to speaking the truth in love?

> Take time this week to practice repeating the "Is that the truth?" question. How many times do you have to typically repeat the question before you get to the really critical truths? How does this iteration of the truth question become your own fierce conversation with yourself?

End Notes:

1. *Cognitive unconscious.* You, like me and everyone else, live in a matrix of meaning frames. Many of these meanings were given to you— you inherited them in the language(s) you learned, in the home you were born into, in your school, religion, culture, etc. Many of these frames you invented with your childhood mind from birth to adulthood as you thought and felt in trying to figure out what life is about, what you are about, what things mean, how they work, what leads to what, etc. Now most of these frames exist within you in your cognitive unconscious. You live in them as you live in the atmosphere; you breathe them in without any awareness of them. Your cognitive unconscious also includes neurological processes in your body and neurology that enables you to see, hear, process information, etc.

2. See the Matrix Model (2003).

3. *Demanding* that you get it just right, that you get it perfectly, that you get it all now will counter the calmness, relaxation, and safety of your Crucible space. These emotions and the frames that drive them, will interfere with being able to effectively use the Crucible as a tool for transformation.

4. *User's Manual of the Brain, Volume II* (1999). *Communication Magic* (2001). Defusing Hotheads and other Cranky People. This training manual is for dealing with people who are at their stress threshold.

5. Cognitive dissonance is the process that changes your mind, attitude, and/or behavior when you experience inner incongruence. For example, you buy something that you had some question about. One part of you believes in it, another doubts. The tension created by the cognitive dissonance predicts that eventually you will either become a believer, feel convinced, or you'll return the item or suffer buyer's remorse?

6. For more about the levels of meaning, see *Unleashed* (2007), the first section.

7. Genesis 33:24-32.

Chapter 11

APPRECIATION

The Sacrilizing Art

*"The highest and last of the characteristics
of self-actualizers is that of continued freshness of appreciation."*
Abraham Maslow

You might think that telling the truth and getting to the heart of your constructed meanings might be the final step in the self-actualizing transformation. Surprise, it is not. More is required.

There must also be love, responsibility, ownership, and integration so in this we're a long way from being done. There are several more requirements. While truth is central, truth alone is not enough. *There must be love*—"truth spoken in love." And the *love* part is not only about the value and awe of the person, it is also about the ability to find value, to create value, to see value, and to speak value. The verb that I am highlighting here is "valuing"—and it is that action that drives the state of *appreciation*.

Ah, *appreciation*. It is about the core competency of *appreciating* that enables you to find your highest truths—your best truths, the noble truths that will transform you from the inside-out. How is that? How does that work? It works due to the fact that inside of *appreciation* is the ability to see, recognize, honor, speak, and create *value*. After all, what do you appreciate if not the very things that you value? And the more you value something, the more you appreciate it. In fact, *to recognize value is to appreciate.* To appreciate is to recognize, detect, create, and confirm value. So, have I made the point? Valuing and appreciating are facets of the same thing, synonyms that describe the same phenomena.

Appreciation refers to positively evaluating the worth and value of something. It is to enjoy and delight in the value of something and to admire because of that value. When you appreciate, you give yourself to the presence of what you value, adoring its preciousness. And this power, this ability of seeing, recognizing, and honoring the value of something is a very special skill. It is to see how a person, event, or an experience can bring richness and benefits, it is to see meaningfulness. Meaningfulness? Yes, because *only that which is meaningful is valuable.* Without meaning, there is no value— nothing to appreciate.

Meaningfulness

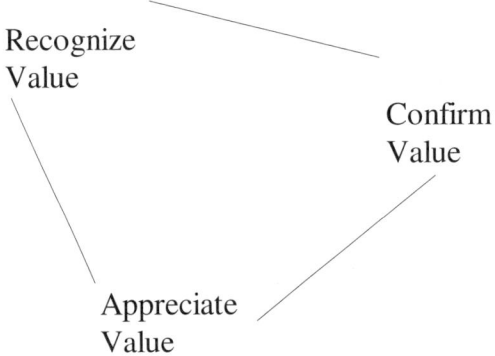

Maslow used a special word for this, a word that many find shocking on first hearing—"sacrilize." In using this, the word *sacred* is used in its sociological sense. Sociologically, sacred refers to distinguishing the value of something in and of itself, for itself, apart from what you can do with it, or how you can use it. *To sacrilize is to see the value of something for itself.* That is, to recognize that thing (a person, object, event, or experience) as an *end value* rather than an *instrumental value.* Or as Maslow often said, "To see it in the light of eternity." And about sacrilizing, he said:

> "*Sacrilizing:* To see a person or event "under the aspect of eternity." To see things as precious, sacred, special, highly significant, and important in and of themselves.

> "This is the most important way of helping a person move toward self-actualization."

Actually we have already encountered appreciation and developed appreciation within the Crucible even if I have not made that explicit before now. When there is an appreciation of another person's point of view and perspective apart from your own, then there is *accurate empathy.* Then, when you have an appreciation of a person's innate value, you see and relate to them with *unconditional positive regard.* And when there is an appreciation of reality, of authenticity, and genuineness, then there is *truth.*

Appreciation gives you magical eyes. In appreciation, you look behind and beyond the surface and discover what's inwardly valuable, important, and meaningful to yourself or another. It takes special kind of eyes to be able to do that. If you only see the surface you will be blind to the value within, the diamonds and gems that lie hidden beyond the surface. When you see beyond the surface to the person's inner value and wonder, you develop a sacrilizing perspective. This brings me to the quotation from Maslow about how the powers and potentials of human nature are so often dampened and inhibited:

> "Every baby has possibilities for self-actualization but most get it knocked out of them. I think of the self-actualizing man not as an ordinary man with something added but rather as *the ordinary man with nothing taken away.* The average man is a human being with dampened and inhibited powers." 1 (Edward Hoffman's biography of Maslow, *The right to be human, 1988,* p. 174)

The problem with fully developing this resource of appreciation is that normally we see only with our physical eyes and not with our deeper or higher eyes for detecting, recognizing, honoring, and articulating hidden value. Yet if you believe in the possibility for self-actualization in every person then you will want to give yourself to *developing the ability to look beyond surface impressions.* You will look for potential value, for possibilities that are still in an embryo state— just the seed of what can be.

In NLP we do this with the operational frame of mind that is summarized in the premise: "Beyond every behavior is a positive intention." Now that positive intention may not occur in the first behavior, or the next behavior, or the one after that, yet if you keep searching, if you keep asking, you will ultimately find a positive intention that began a person's final response. Obviously, this doesn't validate the person's surface behavior that might have been extremely ugly and hurtful. Not at all. But it does enable you to separate person from behavior and to treat the person as more and other than the behavior— which is the point.

Here's another secret about appreciation: Appreciation is the attitude that drives the source of wealth creation. Did you know that? Do I now have your attention? How is that? It's because wealth is created by finding problems that are important enough to solve and that by finding solutions, people would value and will invest their money in.[1]

No wonder entrepreneurs have eyes for both problems and solutions. *Solutions* that do not relate to important problems are useless and valueless. No one would want them, let alone pay for them. But to see and appreciate a problem as worth solving is the first step in seeing an opportunity for finding or creating a solution to it—that describes the eyes of an entrepreneur. And it all begins by embracing a problem with appreciation. Now that's appreciation in a whole new dimension, is it not?[2]

Appreciating Moping Disappointment
Every year I attend the NLP Conference in London and in 2008 I made a presentation on *The Crucible*. During the London conference I demonstrated the use of the Crucible with two participants. Later a middle-age man by the name of James approached me.

> "I was really impressed and touched by the power of the Crucible as a change process when I saw the demonstrations, and I was just about to volunteer, but then felt that the details of my specific situation were too personal. Is there a chance you could do the process with me?"

As circumstances had it that year, I did have a little bit of time in London before flying to Italy, and so I took James on to do the process. "Since you know what the Crucible is and what it is for, we can get right to it. So, what do you want to take into the Crucible?" James explained that he had been experiencing and suffering from a depression that began when he went through a break-up of an intimate relationship. "Okay, so you want to take that relationship into the Crucible?"

> "Yes, and my emotions about that relationship. I would like to take the distress of the breakup and a tremendous disappointment that I've experienced through the whole process of breaking up. I would like to take my depression and all that's involved in that."

As I engaged James in the process, I made sure that he had a Crucible place that brought out his best and that he had each of the elements. That didn't take long since he had heard my presentation, so within twenty minutes we were ready to begin the encounter. I invited him to sit back and to just experience and enjoy his inner space of safety. After a few minutes, I then asked him the beginning question. "Okay, if you are fully ready then I want you to bring in all of your hurting emotions from the breakup into this very special place—your stress and distress, your disappointment and depression, just allow those feelings to come into this place so that you can witness and accept them as the emotions you have experienced about it. And how is that?"

> "It's okay. I don't like it, but it's like I'm observing those emotions rather than being deeply inside them. And I can see myself with them."

"Good. So just witness how you do these emotions, how you create the distress in your mind and heart, how you create the disappointment and depression. Notice what you say to yourself to create these feelings. Notice the words you use, the tone of voice that you use, the pictures and images that you use ... and just notice. Just witness. You are just watching human stuff ... human emotions. And be with that. And how's that?"

> "Hmmmm. It's strange. I had not really noticed the words or imagines or tones that I use when I feel those feelings. It has always seemed that the feelings just came and did a job on me rather than I had any part in it."

"And as you become aware of that, what else are you aware of?"

> "Well, that I play a part in creating my emotions. I hate saying that; it makes me responsible, but I know that that's true anyway."

"Is that your truth, James? Is it true that you are responsible for your emotions and that you play a role in creating them? Is that your truth?"

> "Yes. That's my truth. ... [long pause]."

"And so what will you now *do* about that?"

> "*Do* about that? Uhhhhh. I guess I have to take responsibility for my emotions, but I don't know what else to do about that."

"James, what have you been doing with your emotions? What actions or non-actions, what behaviors, what responses—inward or outward, have you engaged in given the emotions of distress, disappointment, and depression?"

> "Oh. Well, I've been moping around a lot, I've been dis-engaging in the things that I used to do that I enjoyed, and I've been angry, really angry ... at myself and at others, at her! And I have been lashing out, I guess I have been returning pain for pain. ... [Pause] ... I have been doing a lot of blaming, and I'm ashamed to say that I became physically aggressive toward her on a couple of

occasions."

"And as you *witness* what you just said, and just *accept* that that's been some of what's happened, recognizing the actions that came out of the old meanings and old emotions, what will you now *do* as you take responsibility for creating the emotions?"

> "I'll stop all of those things. I will stop moping around; that has really undermined everything. It's made me act like a spoiled brat wanting ... no, demanding the world serve me."

"Is that your truth? That moping around about things has really undermined everything turning you into a spoiled brat having a tantrum?"

> "Yes! That is really true. I can't believe that I didn't see that before."

"So what new behaviors will you take *responsibility to do that will replace the old behaviors*?"

> "I will *not* mope! That's for sure. I will stop that."

"Good. That sounds pretty definite. And if you are not moping around, what will you be doing?"

> "Hmmmm." [Long pause]

"James, allow yourself now to move over to your *appreciation* lookout in your special space ... and as you move there and access your ability to see value and appreciate, what can you appreciate about all of this and what can you appreciate about ..."

> "Oh, yes! I can appreciate the warning power of disappointment! [giggling] Disappointment is like a wake up call shouting at me to check out my expectations, and especially the demands I put on myself and others, and to move from demanding and blaming to appreciating."

"That sounds pretty life changing ..."

> "Yes! I now know what I did that really messed up the relationship—I failed to appreciate Belinda as I wanted to and as she needed."

"James, is that your truth?"

> "Yes, I said I loved her, but I actually failed to love her practically because I didn't appreciate her. [Nervous giggling and wiping away tears.] And the sad thing is that I never realized that; not until now.

And because I didn't, I blamed her and got angry and aggressive, and I didn't need to get defensive at all."

"So your truth is what? What truth have you discovered that is now setting you free from the distress, the disappointment, and the depression?"

"My truth is—*True love appreciates!* My truth is that it was my demands and unrealistic expectations that set me up, and her up, and us up, so that I failed to truly love. My truth is that I will use disappointment as a warning signal and I will focus on finding the good and the valuable in everything instead of acting selfish and self-centeredly in blaming others."

Appreciate by Endowing with Richer Meanings
The quality of your life is a function of the quality of our meanings.[3] Is that a surprising realization? Or do you already know that? And if the quality of your life and meanings are so interrelated, then to enrich the quality of your life, the first step is to take ownership of the meanings that you create and attribute to things. Do that and you can then operate from richer and more robust meanings, meanings that will enable you to appreciate things at a much higher level.

The skill that drives appreciation is the competence of being able to create rich meanings at will, to take charge of your meaning-making skills. Are you ready to develop, use, and expand your powers for constructing rich and robust meanings? The design of the following process is to enable you to develop a resilient mind that can quickly and efficiently create rich and robust meanings. It is to discover and develop your own innate ability to create meaning and to extend your creative meaning-making.

Accessing Appreciation
Have you ever melted in appreciation? What caused that? What was the trigger for that state and experience of appreciation? To develop this capacity, make a list of all the things you have or could appreciate. When you have completed your list, keep it with you for a full month and keep recording big and little appreciations. By then you will probably gather a hundred items or more. [Yes, 100!] After that you can continue your *appreciation search* by asking friends and colleagues for their list of things that they appreciate.

Once you have a pretty good list, go through it and find your top five. What are the top five things that you appreciate— something that when you think about it, you begin to melt in appreciation? Now test it. Does it work?

How well does it work? How much can you melt in appreciation by turning your thoughts and emotions to that item? What is your number one item for inducing appreciation?

> *The quality of your life is a function of the quality of our meanings.*

The funny thing about appreciation is that the best examples tend to be the simplest things—a smile, a touch, a special moment, a word of encouragement. As you find your top five, practice going into an appreciative state with each and begin to notice how you do it, and what it is like when you fully experience it? Gauge the intensity of the appreciation from 0 to 10. How easily can you now access a state of appreciation, at a level of 8 or 9? In this state, how do you breathe, what is your posture, how do you look out at the world with the eyes of appreciation? Be sure to set an anchor for this state.

Unlike acceptance, appreciation is a very warm and emotional state. Here you are welcoming something into your world, and you are doing so with joy, with passion, with the delight of knowing and feeling that it is valuable. Appreciation is an especially optimistic state as it registers the things that make life good and precious. No wonder appreciation is a key ingredient for living with vitality.

Appreciation Blocks
Did you have any problems with accessing an intensive state of appreciation? A great many people do. In fact, I think that it tends to be an occupational hazard of high achievers. How does that work? Why would a high achiever *not* appreciate or block appreciation? Simple, by discounting. In pursuit of excellence, today's accomplishments are downgraded and discounted as nothing. The passion for more, to be better, keeps one from fully appreciating today's accomplishments. Given this let's flush out any and every appreciation block. What are the blocks to appreciation? What could interfere with and dampen your ability to appreciate? There are quite a number of things. Here is a short list of the key factors:

1) Getting used to blessings: taking things for granted.
2) Continually raising your standards and expectations.
3) Discounting: the failure to let something count, treating it as a nothing.
4) Over-focusing on your next goals.
5) Impatience: not taking the time to count, to savor the value of the things that you do have or have created.

The Meanings that Drive Appreciation
If meaning is the inner factor of value and appreciation, then the factor that cleanses your truths, that relives it in the fires of the Crucible is your twin-abilities to *first suspend low level meanings and then create rich and robust meanings at higher levels.* If you value what you find meaningful, the more meaning you can bring to anything, to the smallest of things, the more meaningful it will feel, the more value and so the more you can appreciate it— the more you love.

Conversely, the less meaning you bring to something—the less meaningful it will be, the less value it will have to you, the less appreciation you will feel. That's why ultimately appreciation is a function of your powers of meaning making, a function of your ability to find value in things.

Crucible Coaching
In your notebook, *My Transformational Life,* devote a page to "Things I Appreciate." And this week begin your list of things that you appreciate. After all, if appreciation is the state and skill that in itself is a value-creating activity, where will you start as you begin to develop your capacity for appreciation?

One of the things that can hold you back from this is the fear that "appreciating" will make you weak or soft or that it will make you vulnerable to disappointment. So check it out.

> Do you have full permission within yourself to simply *appreciate*? If not, then take time to give yourself permission to add this capacity to your repertoire. How many meanings can you create that will support this ability? Take time this week also to make a list of the meanings that you will give to appreciating so that you become a world-class appreciator.

> Did you stop and do the appreciation accessing process? If not, plan to access some referents that easily and powerfully put you into a state of appreciation. As you do that, take time to take a snapshot of what *appreciation* feels like, and what it does to you in your body. As you become more and more familiar with this powerful state, set a trigger so that you can "anchor" this state and have more ready accessibility to it.

End of Chapter References

1. *Inside-Out Wealth* (2010). See Chapter 5 on the Best Meanings for Wealth Creation and "the heart of wealth."

2. This is the theme of the third Self-Actualization Workshop, *Unleashing Creative Solutions.*

3. The quality of your life is the quality of your states, your meanings is one of the key points in the Meta-States Model. See *Secrets of Personal Mastery* (1999).

Chapter 12

RESPONSIBILITY

The Power of Response

"That we are free to think or not to think, and to live responsibly or irresponsibly, reflects the essence of what it means to be human. This freedom is our burden, our challenge, our glory. ... We create our selves through what we are willing to take responsibility for."
Nathaniel Brandon (1996, p. 56)

"Life ultimately means taking the responsibility to find the right answer to its problems and to fulfill the tasks which it constantly sets for each individual."
Viktor Frankl (1959, p. 122)

"Your first responsibility is to be yourself honestly and fully."
Abraham Maslow (1996, p. 67)

I noted at the beginning of the last chapter that truth is not enough. Love is certainly needed—the ability to love and care about what you value and find meaningful, which is why I added *appreciation* to the Crucible in the last chapter. Now for the next one—*ownership*—the ability to own with full responsibility your truth, your valuing, your highest meanings.
• What does it take in order to assume ownership of your responses so that you fully recognize your power to respond?
• What is required for a person to become a response-able person?

From the exploration into the elements of the Crucible, we know that it takes ego-strength, unconditional positive regard for your value and worth, a strong sense of appreciation for your powers, and an appreciation of your fundamental powers to speak and live the truth. Truth and truth-telling lies at the core because truth sets us free enabling us to become real—authentic. Yet there's more.

The Semantically Loaded Word
If there's any word that is semantically loaded, *responsibility* has to be at the top of the list. I mis-used the word once. I had taken a contract to work with boys 14 to 18 years of age who were in a lock-up situation. These boys had all been involved in violent crimes and the Department of Corrections in Colorado wanted them to learn responsibility. So that was my objective. But I made a mistake. My mistake was that I walked in on the first day and wrote the word *responsibility* on the white board. I did that because I wanted to start a life-changing conversation with them. To say that such was not the way to do it is an tremendous understatement.

Well, you can imagine how well that went over! It didn't. I saw a couple of the boys put their index finger in their mouth pretending to gag! Their attitude as they told me later was,
> *"Responsibility— why in the world would we want that? That's never gotten us anything or anywhere! It's only brought us trouble and pain."*

I explored with the group of boys what they thought about "responsibility." I discovered that, to them, the word already held powerfully negative meanings—what it meant to them was "trouble," "blame," "pain," "punishment." No wonder they didn't want to learn how to be responsible! No wonder they knew I was an idiot! The word was semantically loaded with some of the most painful emotional states possible. No wonder they treated it as they did tests and summer school!

The next week I returned and wrote the word *response power* on the white board. "Who would like to have response-*power*?" I asked emphasizing the word *power*. "Who would like the *power* to make the response you want to make and to choose your response so that you make powerful responses that serves you well over the long

> "We who lived in concentration camps can remember the men who walked through the huts comforting others, giving away their last piece of bread ... they offer sufficient proof that everything can be taken from a man, but one thing: the last of the human freedoms—to choose one's attitude in any given set of circumstances, to choose one's own way."
> Viktor Frankl
> *Man's Search for Meaning* (p. 102)

term?" Suddenly I had their attention. They wanted *that*! Whew, saved from being an idiot!

Actually this highlights the informative nature of the word response-ability. Literally it refers to *the ability* (the capacity, the competence) *to respond* to things. And when we break down this ability, it to comes down to your most basic responses or powers of thinking, emoting, speaking, and behaving. These are your most fundamental powers.[1] No matter what happens, you can always make a mental response, an emotional response, a verbal or linguistic response, and a behavioral response.

Response-ability
The essential idea within *responsibility* is that of power, energy, vitality, ownership, proactivity, and taking initiative. Given all of that, who would be against that? Who would resist any of that? And yet we do. And not just a few of us, we all do. We resist because it is easier to complain. It is easier to "explain why" we can't do something, why something is too much, too hard, will take too much energy, money, etc. It is much easier to blame and to find fault with others. Ah, here we see the opposite of responsibility —*playing helpless.* If you are not taking responsibility, you are playing the victim—thinking, feeling, and acting as if you lack the power to respond as you would like to.

What else are you doing when you are *not* taking responsibility? You are making excuses. You are excusing yourself from action and from making a response that makes a difference. You are whining or complaining or focusing on objections and using your intelligence perversely to excuse yourself from excellence, from your vision, and from your highest and best.

And this will come up whenever you enter into the Crucible! Expect it. Expect that you, and those that you facilitate through the process, will make excuses. Then what? What do you do then? That's when you access and utilize the resource of ownership or responsibility. And you will do that, ask responsibility-evoking questions:
- What is your decision? What will you decide or choose?
- Given this, what will you do?
- What response will you now make when X happens?
- What are you now choosing to think, feel, say, or do?
- What will you do about that symptom?
- What will be your highest and most noble choice?

And if there's any hesitation, then step back to the confrontational challenge

of truth speaking and go for the heart of the matter again— the meanings that you or the other person is creating or utilizing that govern his or her responses.
- So is your truth that you have no choice in this matter?
- So your truth is to excuse yourself from what you really want?
- So you are going to choose to give up?
- Are you, right now, experiencing yourself as an active and prime mover of your world?
- Right now, in the Crucible, are you self-determining your frames?
- If not, are you ready to do that?

The excuses that you'll hear in the Crucible are all of the everyday excuses beginning with the trivial and whinny ones—"It's too hard," "It's too cold," "It takes too long," "I don't have enough money," etc. Then there will be the more existential excuses:
- "That's just the way I am."
- "I feel so guilty, I'm just flawed and sinful."
- "I'm afraid, I don't have the courage to face that."
- "I can't do anything as long as he acts that way; I'm just stuck, always have been, always will be."
- "I chose that and now I just have to live with my choices."

And with each excuse, go right in and confront the response-ability of the person (whether the person is you or someone else). It is at this place in the Crucible where the person's processes will produce a lot of heat and tension. It is the heat of stepping up to choice-point and accepting one of the scariest things in the world—to accept existential responsibility for your life, for your choices, and for your destiny.

Pseudo-Guilt and The Crucible
When I facilitated Jason in his Crucible space, he wanted to confront and deal with a business relationship that had failed. When we got to the heart of things, we discovered that he had not come through on several projects that were his responsibility. "I did wrong; I'm as guilty as hell for doing that."

That seemed pretty definitive, so I asked him, "Is that your truth?" He confirmed that it was, and commented:
"That's just the way it is, I'm guilty."
"So Jason," I said, "Tell me about this guilt. Is this real guilt or is this pseudo-guilt?"
"Well, sure it is real guilt!"

"Okay, so what law did you violate?"

"What? What law ...?" [Pause]

"Well, if you are guilty, then you have broken some law, maybe man's law, a legal misdeed, or maybe God's law, some divine law that you believe in. So what law did you violate?"

"Well, ... I don't know. I didn't violate any law that I can think of, I just failed to come through on the projects, I just procrastinated so long that I lost business for the company."

"So there's no divine law that says, 'Thou shalt always come through on every project you engage in on planet earth!?" So if you didn't break a law and aren't guilty as a law-breaker, then you are just feeling bad for failing to be fully responsible for what you had agreed to do? Is that what's actually true about this situation?"

"Hmmmm. I never thought of it that way before. I just felt really bad and ashamed, and felt so guilty."

"And now?"

"Well, I don't know. I still feel guilty."

"Guilty of ...?"

"Well, I don't know. I just feel bad. I feel really ashamed of myself."

"So is that your truth? That you feel really ashamed of yourself and 'bad' for not following through on what you should have done? [Yes.] So what will you now *do*?"

"Do? I don't know. There's nothing to do. The business is gone and it's my fault."

"And now that you realize that, now that you have come face to face with that truth, *what will be different* from this day forward? What will you do differently when you collaborate with someone? When you make promises and accept a project? What will you choose to *do* from this day forward?"

"But what about the guilt, the bad feelings?"

"What about them? Will you let those feelings stop you from changing? What will you *do* now to make any amends that you need to make to your business partner?"

That was the moment when Jason began to fully *feel* the shame and embarrassment. That's when the tears came and that's when *he stopped using the pseudo-guilt to feel bad without doing something about it* and without changing. Later he commended that it was so uncomfortable being held in that place with his "guilt." He said he was squirming inside with my confrontation and just wanted to get out of there. But he said that the safety of the place as well as my framing, made it possible for him to confront the bad feelings and *feel* them so that he could use them for cleansing and renewal.

Fully Responsible but not Omnipotently Responsible
One challenge of entering into the Crucible is that of fully accepting responsibility for yourself so that you become self-responsible in a healthy and robust way that supports and actualizes your best potentials. To do this will unleash increasingly more of your possibilities and potentials and make you more alive to your unique contributions.

There are some extremes to avoid as you think about responsibility. One extreme is to not overdo it and assume that you are responsible for everything! You are not. Enthusiasts for responsibility have often gone to extremes with this. "I am responsible for everything I create." "I totally create my reality." These ideas are often propagated as by New Age thinkers as evidenced recently in the movie and book, "The Secret."[2] But they are wrong in their grandiosity and extravagant claims. While free will is a force in your life, it is not the only force.

Will Schultz, from the first HPM, took this to incredibly ridiculous extremes. In his book *Profound Simplicity* he repeatedly wrote that "we choose everything in our lives from the beginning" of our lives (page 29). About rape, he argued that most people who are raped somehow have an unconscious wish for it. Did I say that there are incredibly ridiculous extremes?
> "I feel that, in most cases, the rapees have an unconscious wish to collude with the rapist to perform the act of rape. Many rapees would not make such a choice if they were fully aware." (p. 38)

And if that isn't outrageous enough, he then tells the story of a five-year-old daughter of a friend. He had the gall to ask his friend to speak to the young child so that she would "open herself to the possibility that she chose the event and see if that orientation made any sense to her." (p. 38). Without recognizing that every idea has limits, this is the kind of utter stupidity that can result!

The truth is that your responsibility and mine is limited and limited in numerous ways. Why is that and how is it? One thing that creates this is the fact that all of your choices and response-abilities are fallible. That is, they are not infallible and not omnipotent. You could only be absolutely and totally responsible only if you were God— infallible, omnipotent, and omnipresent.[3]

Next, the responsibility that each of us have is limited by how our actions as responses interact with each other. What if several of us try to respond to a person being mugged at the same time and in doing so get in each other's way so that we complicate things and make a mess of our rescue efforts? Or what if a group of people observe someone in need and each assumes that someone else will respond. There's all kind of ways that our responses (and responsibilities) can intermingle. What this means is that most things are over-determined by a great multitude of contributing factors. Things are not so simple as to have one and only one factor that "causes" it. Reality, and especially social relationships, are multi-caused.[4]

Maslow addressed this when he noted that there's a limit to one's responsibility; "one cannot be everything to everybody." Not only that, but "I must allow people their own responsibility." Describing this as a circle of responsibilities, he said that the further the circle extends out from you, the less responsibility you have (1996, p. 67).

Responsibility does not mean blaming. Assuming responsibility has nothing to do with blaming, not even yourself. Instead, *to assume responsibility is to acknowledge a response* that you made and the immediate effect that it has created. You can even acknowledge the responses of others to it—and how they chose to respond or react. Rather than seeking to blame, you would do better to seek to understand how humans respond in interaction with each other's responses.

Blaming, by contrast, is about accusing. It is about getting out your weapon (your index ginger) pointing and making accusations about what others are doing. Yet to do that is to act as if you have no ability or power to chose your responses—which obviously is false. You do have certain powers by which you can respond and that makes you a response-able person.

Actually, it takes "the power to respond" in order to actualize your inner visions into outer performances. That's why responsibility plays such a vital role in the process of actualizing the self as *Abraham Maslow* notes this in the following quotation:
> "Looking within oneself for many of the answers implies taking responsibility. That is in itself a great step toward actualization. . . . In psychotherapy, one can see it, can feel it, can know the moment of responsibility. . . . This is one of the great steps. Each time one takes responsibility, this is an actualizing of the self." (1971, p. 45)

Responsibility For and To

There is a formula for personal success that is as close to *magic* as anything I know for curing some of the most hurtful diseases that afflict humans especially around this element of responsibility. The diseases I'm speaking about are those that infect and weaken our ability to discern reality, create great relationships, and stay sane especially when the world is un-sane. The formula can be summarized using the magic numbers 4-2.

To describe the full story of "responsibility" I'll use the numbers **4-2** as shorthand for two little words—*for* and *to*.[5] These two small words have a great and far reaching impact on your lives as they summarize and convey some of the most important concepts in human experience. The distinction that I'm going after here has to do with your *responses* and so with your *response-abilities*. **4-2** provides a quick way to recognize the difference between what you are *responsible **for*** and who you are *responsible **to***. Doing this creates a powerfully enhancing way to navigate relationships when they can seem more like confusing webs.

It All Begins with Your Responses

Let's begin with *your powers to respond.* No matter what happens, you always can and do respond, and in fact, you always do respond—even if only inwardly. You respond with your mind by thinking about it, representing it, relating it to other things, pondering it, creating ideas and beliefs about it, making decisions, setting frames and understandings about it. All of this relates to the most internal world of your thoughts. And in this private domain, *no one can make you think anything.* Yet they can trigger your thoughts. They can invite you to think in a certain way. But in the end, *your thoughts are your thoughts.* (See Figure 1:1)

Figure 12:1

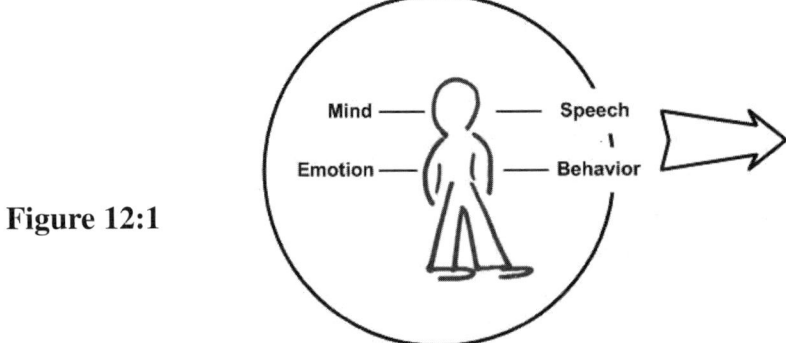

Further, whatever you *think* about something—that thought creates and governs your *feelings* about it. Your feelings, emotions, and moods are also responses. They describe your emotional responses to things. So whatever happens, you are always responding at an emotional level. You feel. And generally, as you think about it, so you will feel. This creates energy, somatic energy, in your body so that you can do something about your thoughts. And while you sometimes regress in times of stress to a more primitive state and say, "You make me angry" or afraid, or jealous, or happy, or whatever, the truth is that *your emotions* like your thoughts are *your emotions.*

Those are your two private powers. And from those responses you have two public powers. Publically and outwardly you can respond with speech and behavior. These are your linguistic and behavioral powers by which you can influence the world and actually do something as part of your response. And again, whatever you say, whatever linguistic skills and competencies you develop and use as part of your response—it is *your* response— your power.

First, the For
There's another critical distinction with all of these personal powers for responding to the things that happen in life. Not only is there the distinction between private and public, there is the distinction between what you are response-able *for* and *to*. The first speaks about *what* you can *do* that comes from out of your area of control and the second speaks about how you use those responses as you give them *to* various people. (See Figure 1:2)

What are you are responsible *for?* I'm sure the answer is obvious. I am responsible *for* the responses that I can make. You are responsible *for* your mental responses (your thoughts), your emotional responses (your feelings), your verbal and behavioral responses (what you say and do). And all of this responsibility *for* describes *accountability.* We ask that you give account for what you do, for your actions, your behaviors, and for all of your responses. If you are not responsible for these things, then who is? This is your area of control.

Responsibility *for* defines and describes the concept of *accountability.* And what is accountability? It is a relationship condition wherein others hold you "to give account" for what you do. If you are in a relationship where you are accountable for something, then you agree, at least in principle, that they can treat you as the person who will invest your actions, behaviors, and responses to get something done. If you do not get it done, then you are responsible in that you are the one wh will give account for the actions or lack of actions and you are the one who will have to do something to make up for it.

So imagine yourself inside a sphere—a bubble of energy that extends throughout to your personal sense of space, perhaps the length of your arms (so a yard or meter out and all around you). This is your area of accountability. Let's think of it as your response zone or your power zone, your power bubble. Within it arise your thoughts, feelings, words, and actions. You generate these from within and so they arise and come from out of you. Nobody outside the circle can be responsible *for* these responses, they are ours.

Moving on out to the *To*
The tiny little word *to* describes *relationships*. By your public powers of speech and behavior you *relate to* people, groups, teams, organizations, etc. and so when you are *responsible to* someone or a group, this creates all kinds of relationship: familial, friendship, cultural, career, governmental, and so on. These are the systems that you live in and the persons, groups, and communities to whom you answer. If you imagine an arrow that moves out from the circle of your power zone to others in a larger circle of loved ones, colleagues, friends, etc., that arrow identifies who you are responsible *to*.

Your *for* tells about the what—*the content* of what you think and feel and then outwardly say and do. The *to* speaks about *the context* of the persons with whom you offer these personal responses.

Figure 12:2

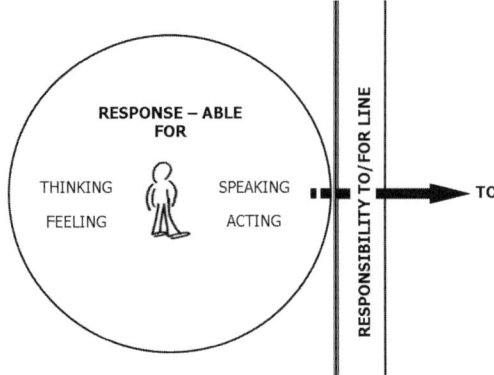

And Now — The Line
Let's now draw a *line* to separate and distinguish *relationship* (responsibility to) and *accountability* (responsibility for). Draw this line so that you can distinguish two kinds of responses that you make. First identify a response *for* whatever it is that you are thinking, feeling, saying, and doing, and then we identify *to* whom you are making this response.

The sanity rule here is simple to understand, but very difficult to put into action. It is this:
> You are *only* response-able *for* the responses that you generate mentally, emotionally, verbally, and behaviorally. Your ability to respond (responsibility) ends at your nose or the edge of the reach of your arm. You cannot be responsible *for* much that goes on beyond this line.

Similarly, when you set the frame that you have lots of relationships that set up various accountabilities and inter-relational dynamics, then you realize that there are numerous people, situations, and groups *to whom* you live in a responsible relationship.

The first distinction (*responsibility for*) enables you to access your *inner game of personal power.*[5] Highlighting your four powers (thinking, emoting, speaking, and behaving) you circumscribe your "power zone" and give it a definite area with boundaries. You define where and how you can respond and what lies beyond that area. As you then focus on and develop these functions within this zone, you *empower* yourself. When you focus on things outside this zone, responses that belong to others, you *dis-empower* yourself.

The second distinction of *responsibility to* focuses your attention on the exchanges you negotiate with others as you step into, and out of, relationships. In your interactions with others, what you give and receive are the external responses of speech and behavior. It is what you say and how you say it with your actions that you use to negotiate with. When you negotiate, you ask that another person speaks and behaves to you in certain ways. Making these distinctions clarifies roles and relationships and so enhances sanity, that is, a good adjustment to social and inter-personal reality. A consequence of this is that it reduces your stress. It enables you to navigate the waters of inter-dependency with others and to avoid the shoals of co-dependency.

So the central rule for winning this inner game[6] that will empower you

personally and enable you to know precisely where your control ends and your influence begins is the following:
- When you focus on your power zone, you empower yourself.
- Conversely, when you focus outside of this zone, you dis-empower yourself.

It is that simple; it is that profound. Being independent enables you to know and own your own response-abilities, assume complete responsibility *for* yourself (for what you think, feel, say, and do), and assume responsibility *to* others. When you are independent you can easily share your independence with another because you recognize and accept that relationships are conditional.

Relationship as Responsibility *To* Another
Responsibility to creates and defines your interactions and relationships. If I am responsible *to* you, then my relationship with you is defined in terms of those responses that I give *to* you. The responses that I promise, or that are understood as belonging to the relationship—these responses define the relationship.

If I ask a friend what he would like from me, he might say that he wants me to meet him for a jog by the river trail. So we agree upon a time and place. When I come through by responsibly acting in a way so that I give him what he asked for and what I said I would do, I have been responsible. I have been responsible *to* him *for* what we agreed with him that I would do. When I do not do what I said, then I don't come through, on my promises. I have not been responsible. Now I need to make it right by communicating or apologizing or in some way showing that it matters to me that I failed to carry through on my side of the agreement and acknowledge how it has negatively affected him and our relationship.

If every relationship can be understood, defined, and even analyzed in terms of the actions we promise to give *to* each other, then we can ask questions to identify how we want to shape our relationships.
- How would you like for me to talk to you?
- What tone or volume would you like me to use when I'm upset?
- What would you like for us to do together as a couple?
- What counts for you as an enjoyable evening out?
- What counts for you in the giving and receiving of affection?

Relationship emerges from these sets of actions that we *give to* and *receive from* each other. In the best of healthy relationships we joyfully accept that we are responsible *to* each other. We're thrilled to respond to each other and we make things right when we haven't been fully responsible to each other.

All relationships operate in this way. Even business relationships involve a set of actions that you have said that you will give *to* your employer to get the things that you want (employment, pay, benefits, opportunities, etc.). This *giving and receiving* dimension of relating with each other defines the quality of the relationship.

The inside dimension of your responses are your thoughts and feelings. What you think and feel is what makes you responsive or not-responsive to the other person. This area also generates your attitudes, dispositions, moods, and beliefs which then temper, qualify, and condition the "feel" for how you do what you do as you relate to another person. In healthy relationships you are responsive, caring, respective, supportive, open, vulnerable, etc. Frequently you find yourself feeling these emotions, but unskilled or unable to translate these into effective behaviors that accurately transmit them. This is where you relate to your loved one by asking them what counts and even inviting them to coach you into how to behave in ways that count for love, or respect, or care to them.

Relationships, as composed of *the sets of interactions,* give you a hands-on understanding of what you are specifically giving and receiving from each other. Amazing words— those two small words "to" and "for" — are they not? Each small word gives a different concept—concepts which are critically involved in understanding relationships. Your *to* and *for* responses identify accountability and then relationship. Both emerge from your *responses* and yet both create very different experiences.

The 4-2 Formula and the Crucible
When you know *what* you are responsible *for* and accept it, you take a big step to sanity, to clarity, and to effectiveness. Similarly, when you know the persons with whom you relate you take another significant step forward toward personal success. Now you can clearly define the responses that you are responsible for, the responses you are to give *to* them. Then you can determine if you have a healthy or unhealthy relationship or an inter-dependent one or a co-dependent one. As you now take care to make these unique distinctions you develop the ability to use responsibility as another aspect of unleashing potentials.

Maslow speaks of responsibility as being an active and creative center in

yourself:
> "The person in peak experience feels himself to be the responsible, active, creative center of his activities and his perceptions. He is now most free of blocks, inhibitions, cautions, fears, doubts, controls, reservations, self-criticisms, etc. He is most spontaneous, more expressive, more innocently behaving, more natural. He is more creative." (p. 106)
>
> "Your first responsibility is to be yourself honestly and fully. This little formula condenses many other formulas as well as encompasses the concepts of self-actualization, inner growth, and the like. What it amounts to is the acceptance of reality, the principles of reality, and the acting upon of reality. So even if I am born a paraplegic, I can still be an agent rather than a pawn." (1996, p. 67)

Your Crucible Conversation
The confrontation of responsibility will generate lots of heat and pressure when you simply ask about such. Your awareness of this will help you navigate this facet of the Crucible. It will help you to avoid being burned or attacked.

Crucible Story
Jon told me that his negative emotions had built up and were "festering like an embedded sliver in the flesh of his emotions." So what was going on? A co-worker, Frank had outranked him at work, and repeatedly would call him, "stupid!" and would do so in front of others. For Jon this was intolerable, but his style was to stuff his emotions and try his best to "be nice and not cause trouble." His words were:
> "I could never tell him to shut up or back off, I could never discharge my hurt and anger lest I lose my job or ruin my reputation with others. I wanted to punish him, but he had superiority."

But as you can guess, eventually the stuffing of his emotions built up until he began to react and to over-react. He said that:
> "It was like a deep hurt that was creating a furious anger so that any suggestion about me having an inferior intelligence, I would explode. I simply could not stand to be called stupid. I refused to allow anyone to assassinate my intelligence in that way."

When I then invited Jon into his Crucible, I asked him about his truth. "What is your truth about all of this Jon?"
> "That Frank is evil! That he is the one at fault and should stop it. My life would be great if he would leave ... or change."

"So at this moment in time, that's your truth? [Yes!] Anything else?"
"Yes, Frank is a low-life, garbage head, he is malicious."
"Okay, and anything else?"
"Well, just that some people are unredeemable."
"Okay, and anything else?"
"No, that's about it."
"Good. So Jon, would you summarize your truths then for me?" And he did. Almost word-for-word, he repeated what he just said. And he did so with a lot of emotion. It seemed to me that he had downloaded enough, so I then said the following:

"Now Jon there's something I want you to do, and you may find it challenging, but do so as best as you can. Are you ready? Okay, so now step back and I want you to witness the truths you have just stated and to do so in your Crucible, in your safety zone where you can just witness while maintaining your unconditional self-worth and your ability to just accept life on its own terms, and now what are you aware of?"

[After a long pause.] "I'm aware that I'm doing a lot of blaming. I'm realizing that I'm not taking responsibility for my part in all of that."

"Good, and is that also your truth?"

"Yes. And my truth is also that I've been speaking out of my pain and hurt, and I have been using those words to hurt back as I feel that I've been hurt. And ... also that I am now ready to assume responsibility for my part and see what I can do to change me."

Crucible Coaching

Coaching time! So, do you have full permission to assume and own your own "responses" as your own?

If not, then give yourself that permission until you get the cue from your mind-body system of "Of course!" That will indicate that the permission has taken and is fully incorporated.

Now in your notebook, *My Transformative Life,* devote a page to "Responsibility To and For."

Are you willing to draw the *responsibility for — to* line? Do you know how to draw it in thought, in emotion, in speech, and in behavior? Where in life do you tend to not draw the line or draw the line far into someone else's area of response? Take time this week to practice drawing this line in your language patterns.

If there is a particular relationship that you find that this is particularly hard or difficult, then make a list of the responses that you are willing and able to give to the person. Make it as extensively as you can. Then make a list of the responses that you want the other person to give to you. Once you have the two lists, then go through and check them. Are all of the responses that you give and that you want *behavioral*? That is, are all of them something that you or the other person can *say* or *do*? If not, cross it out. Are you actually able to make these verbal and behavioral responses? Is the other person actually able to make the verbal and behavioral responses you want? If so, does the other person know that such responses are what you *want*? If not, then set up a time to present this to that person.

End Notes

1. The four powers is the Power Zone in Neuro-Semantics and is highlighted in the APG training. Also see *Secrets of Personal Mastery* (1999), *Achieving Peak Performance* (2009).

2. Article, "The Secret of the Secret," see www.neurosemantics.com.

3. And if, as God, you gave man true "freedom of choice" then you are not responsible for what those fallible creatures choose, they are. So even if you're God, you're not absolutely responsible, but share it with other creatures.

4. The story of Kitty Genovese comes to mind. She was the young woman who was the victim in 1964 of being stabbed to death in Queens (New York City). Genovese was chased by an assailant and attacked three times on the street, over the course of thirty minutes, as thirty-eight of her neighbors watched from their windows. Yet during that time, none of these people called the police. Each assumed someone else would!

5. The numbers "four and two" in English sound like the prepositions words *for* and *to*. This will to translate in other languages.

6. The language of *inner* game and *outer* game refers to a metaphor we use in Neuro-Semantics. See *Winning the Inner Game* (2007).

Chapter 13

JOYOUS LOVE

Peaking Out of the Crucible

"We fear our highest possibilities ... we are generally afraid to become that which we can glimpse in our most perfect moments, under the most perfect conditions, under conditions of greatest courage. We enjoy and even thrill to the godlike possibilities we see in ourselves in such peak moments. And yet we simultaneously shiver with weakness, awe, and fear before these very same possibilities."
                    Abraham Maslow (1971: 34)

How do you know that your experience in the Crucible has worked? How do you know that you have succeeded in unleashing new potentials, developing new competencies, and bringing out your highest and best? How would you know? What can you measure to determine that? The answer is both simple and complex:

You become more of who you are—and more alive. You experience the energy and aliveness of your uniqueness and that puts you in touch with your passion and purpose. Vitality is the sign.

This means that the last element of the Crucible is not one that you have to intentionally activate as you do with the other elements. This one arises or emerges from the process. It occurs as an effort or consequences from all of the other activities. It occurs from finding and speaking your truths, from appreciating, and from assuming responsibility. This element differs from the other elements in that *it is a sign that,* within the Crucible, *you have taken a significant step in self-actualizing.*

Suddenly or slowly, whether within or after the Crucible experience *you find yourself falling in love with life in a fresh and joyous way.* You find a genuine joy in giving yourself to a certain passion that fits with your vision and values. You find your vision for how and why to live your life. You wake up with a renewed vitality. And when that happens, you have what we call *a peak experience*—an ecstasy of joy and love, a sense of transcendence.

De-Mystifying the Peak Experience
When I have mentioned the phrase "peak experience" as I travel around and speak about self-actualization, I notice that it typically evokes some curious responses. Some people start blinking ferociously and go into a new age trance (!). Others seem to have a gag responses as if I have just introduced the ultimate superstition. Yet others get excited as if I have just touched on the very secret of life— of being fully alive. So many responses!

What is a peak experience? And how can you use it to detect that you have unleashed some new potentials and moved into the zone of actualizing your highest meanings into your best performances? What is the peak experience that validates your experience in the Crucible?

1) First, a peak experience of self-actualization is an experience of meaning.
Maslow noted this in the following:
> "Life has to have meaning. It has to be filled with moments of high intensity that validate life and make it worthwhile. Otherwise the desire to die makes sense. If there were no joy in life, it would not be worth living. Unfortunately many people never experience joy, those all-too-few moments of total life-affirmation which we call peak experiences." (1971: p. 180)

Where you find meaning in what you are doing, you will find joy as well. They go together. Meaning and joy; joy and meaning. This actually gives us a clearer understanding of human happiness—it is not about pleasure or mere lower need gratification, it is about discovering meaning and creating a meaningful life. The challenge will be to find your own unique version of what's meaningful to you.

And even more synergizing (or not), it will often arise from the ashes of your biggest struggles. That is, out of the very things that have proven the most challenging, you'll often find the most meaningfulness. That will transpire when you have discovered how to solve the questions of life that have driven and engaged you. Into that problem you have invested a lot of yourself—so in finding a solution you'll experience meaningfulness and joy.
> "These are also the 'highest' values in the sense that they come most often to the best people, in the best moments, under the best

conditions. They are the definitions of the higher life, of the good life, of the spiritual life." (1971: p. 105)

In peak experiences something is awakened in you— something very deep that gives you a strong sense of significance and value and love. It not only awakens you, but excites you as an inner force within your heart or your core giving you a big reason for your life, for unleashing more and more of your potentials.

2) Second, the self-actualizing peak experience involves a mind-emotion richness.
> "Is it possible to reach a peak experience through suffering? We have found that the peak experience contains two components—an emotional one of ecstasy and an intellectual one of illumination." (Maslow, 1971, p. 184)

Your peak experience will involve both some cognitive intentionality of your experience—how you do something, how you describe your experience, etc. and that will give you an inner thrill. You may not understand how you can feel an excitement so intensely about what you do —yet you do.

This was what Viktor Frankl discovered in his horrendous concentration camp experiences. In writing about finding an unique meaning of life in that context, Frankl talked about his interpretation of what it means and that when it is an ennobling meaning, then it does not traumatize.
> "It looks as if any experience of real excellence, of real perfection, of any moving toward the perfect justice or toward perfect values tends to produce a peak experience. ... The love of the body, awareness of the body, and a reverence of the body—these are clearly good paths to peak experiences." (1971: 169, 170)
> "Suffering ceases to be suffering in some way at the moment it finds meaning..." (*Man's Search for Meaning,* p. 179)

3) Third, the self-actualizing peak experience involves the resolution of problems.
> "Mathematics can be just as beautiful, just as peak-producing as music. . . If one works with great creators, great scientists, the creative scientists, *that* is the way they talk. The picture of the scientist must change, and is giving way to an understanding of the creative scientist, and the creative scientist lives by peak experiences. He lives for the moments of glory when a problem solves itself . . . the moments of revelation, of illumination, insight, understanding, ecstasy." (1971: p. 171)

There's almost nothing more pleasurable, more ecstatic, more growth producing, as the experience of solving problems. What explains this? I think that, in part, this arises because we humans are by nature problem-solvers. It's our nature to think and contemplate what's not working and to then invent solutions to make it work. That's why when you happen upon a solution to a problem you've been working on, you become thrilled, ecstatic, and joyful. It can initiate a love of life response. You shout, "Eureka!" You may even get so excited that you will jump out of your bathtub and run naked into the street shouting, "Eureka!"

Such happiness arises as a result of the solution. It comes in various forms. Sometimes as a sudden burst of energy and realization, sometimes as a burst of laughter, a sudden surprise or even shock, a relief as it discards a great burden. Yet however it comes, it provides a new lease on life.

If it is in sports, it may be pushing yourself to reach a new level of competency. If it is in business, it could be finding a way to solve a problem in manufacturing, marketing, or management. The problem you solve could be as small as resolving a squeaky door or as big as creating a foundation for hunger in a particular area. It is not the size of the problem that counts, it is the joy of the resolution. That's why it is in the context of problems that you will often find the context for a peak experience. [Ah, did I just present one of the key secrets of self-actualization?][1]

4) Fourth, the self-actualizing peak experience is a little taste of ecstasy, of paradise.

This is why peak experiences are so readily and universally connected and related to "spirituality." For a moment, you transcend yourself, your world, time, context, body, etc., when that happens you will typically find that you lack the words for describing what's happening. You may have an oceanic feeling and feel connected with everything—with everyone—with the universe— with God.

So what is this? I certainly don't know. Yet the mystery and wonder of this is so universal, that it led Maslow to conclude that it is a biological drive and potential within our very nature as humans. It is a potential within our neurology at a biological level. What's even more important is that when you experience it, you feel inspired and elevated. You feel connected to something or someone bigger and more than yourself.

The peak experience is primarily a sign—a sign that you have moved to a higher level of drive. Your drives now are cleansed, purified, and made unselfish. You want to give back, contribute, and make a difference in the world. And when you experience this you are living in the B-drives. This further explains why self-actualization is not about you. It comes through you, yes. Yet ultimately, it is not about you.

Eliciting Peak Experiences
You say that you never have had a peak experience? Maslow discovered this also in his studies, that many people claim to have never experienced a peak experience. At least, it was not labeled such experiences and so they did not think about their experiences in that way. This led him to begin to ask the following to facilitate people in recovering peak experiences. And what he found was that by planting this question, and inquiry, people began noticing and recalling peak experiences.

> "I would like you to think of the most wonderful experience or experiences of your life; happiest moments, ecstatic moments, moments of rapture, perhaps from being in love, or from listening to music or suddenly 'being hit' by a book or a painting, or from *some great creative moment*. First list these. And then try to tell me how you feel in such acute moments, how you feel differently from the way you feel at other times, how you are at the moment a different person in some ways." (1968, *Toward a Psychology of Being,* p. 71)

You can now use these peak experiences for cultivating the very qualities of self-actualizing people.

> "Any person in any of the peak experiences takes on temporarily many of the characteristics which I found in self-actualizing individuals. That is, for the time they became self-actualizers." (1968, p. 97)
>
> "People in peak experiences are most their identity; closest to their real selves, most idiosynergetic, unique, most alive and vital. Here discovery is at a maximum, and inventions at a minimum. More integrated than at other times, less fighting against self, more at peace with self." (1968, p. 104)

Letting the Love of Ecstatic Joy Emerge
As you use the Crucible to "speak the truth in love" to yourself and others you get to the heart of things, and as you do there usually arises a "fire in the belly." That is, you will begin to discover your passions —what you truly care about as you get past your defenses, you find that the ways you have covered up, denied, and refused to face the truth evaporate. And when it does, it leaves a new fire burning within.

How will you know when this has happened? And how will you be able to facilitate this aspect of the Crucible? The answer is actually very simple—ask.

"Given this truth that you now own and appreciate, how do you feel? What's emerging within you because of it? Are you now experiencing a new level of passion or excitement or joy?"

Crucible Coaching
With your notebook, *My Transformative Life*, devote one or two pages to "Peak Experiences," one page for past peak experiences that you will recall and use for learning, and the second one for future peak experiences.

Now make a list of as many peak experiences that you can recall. Use Maslow's elicitation process described in this chapter. Continue to fill in the list for a couple of weeks; notice when those little special moments occur in your life today. When you have completed the list, look at it for patterns. What insights does your life provide you?

Now as you seek to actualizing your highest and best, use your peak experiences to discover what you are truly good at, what excites you, what natural dispositions and talents that are yet only in potentiality that you could turn into a skill. When you find that, the adventure begins.

Do you have full permission to experience the delightful joy of the goodness of life? Check that out and, if not, then give yourself that permission until it completely settles in you.

End of the Chapter References
1. See *Unleashed!* (2007), Chapter 20 "Capitalizing Problems."

PART III

TRANSFORMATION

IN THE CRUCIBLE

Chapter 14

THE CRUCIBLE TRANCE

Patterns for Entering the Crucible

There are general processes that can generate a crucible experience, many natural processes that arise in life. If you want to be intentional, mindful, and systematic in your approach, you will want to identify and use a specific pattern to create a crucible. And the good news is that there are specific patterns for this.

This chapter contains three such patterns. The first pattern is designed so that you can *construct a Crucible* and the second one is for you to *use a Crucible* for transformations. With the first one, it is important to *not use it* while you are creating it. Use the pattern to design and create a Crucible space that will be uniquely safe and empowering for you. When it is complete and ready, then you'll be fully ready for the second pattern when you will actually use the Crucible process for transformation.

The third pattern is designed so that you can identify previous crucible experiences that you've had in your life but did not recognize as crucible experiences and did not use for transformation. But now you can.

While it is possible for you to do this by yourself, especially if you had some form of experiential self-development training, I highly recommend that you have a trained person to facilitate the process with you. That will allow you to more fully experience it and to more fully feel the power of someone holding the space for you.

#1 Crucible Construction Pattern
The design of this pattern is to create your own personal Crucible space for

transformation. While you are describing and putting the crucible together, *do not* use the Crucible for anything. *This pattern is only to create the sacred space.* This process will be easier if you have someone coach you through it by asking the questions and supporting you as you create an inner space that will serve as a transformative Crucible for yourself.

The Pattern
1) Choose a Metaphorical place.
> Where is a place that when you are there, or even when you just think about it, that place brings out the best in you? Where do you go or could you go that would enable you to feel fully alive?
> Would that be a powerful metaphor for your crucible space?
> What metaphor would give that place the qualities to make it rich, robust, and compelling for you?
> Does this place allow space for you, does it allow you to breathe, to explore, to be, and to feel completely safe?
> Menu list:
>> In the presence of someone who unconditionally loves you.
>> In the sacred space of love, oneness, wholeness, safety, reflection, transformation.
>> Light, mountain, beach, lake, chapel, cathedral, mosque, middle of the universe, bubble, golden space, Buddha tree, etc.
>
> Access your special place and imaginatively go there to see, hear, feel, and smell that place. Do so as vividly as you can.

2) Self-Esteem — Unconditional Positive Regard
> How do you best distinguish your *self as a person* from what you *do* as your expressions? As you do this, put it in your special space. Now three questions to elicit *esteem:*
>> What do you esteem as having ultimate value?
>> What's your highest and most sacred value?
>> What elicits a sense of awe and wonder in you?
>
> When you access it and stay with that feeling for a moment, letting it grow and expand throughout your whole neurology, how does it feel when you apply it to yourself as a human being with incredible potentials? How do you feel with this?
> Now fully feel your unconditional value as a person as you consider this specific unleashing of your potentials from whatever has held you back to what you dream about unleashing, how is that?
> Where do you want to put this in your crucible place? How do you represent it so that when you go there you "know" that this resource

is there in your inner world?

3) *Witnessing — Pure Awareness without Judgment*

Have you ever stepped out onto a balcony to look over a street two or three or more stories below? What was it like when you were above things at a distance that allowed you to *just observe*?

How does it feel in your body when you have stepped back into a know-nothing inquisitive state of just witnessing? How *open* do you feel now to just observe and see what's happening?

Are you able to be *next* to it (above it, behind it) without being *in* it? When you get this feeling of witnessing or observing, where do you want to put this in your crucible place? How do you represent it so that when you go there you "know" that this resource is there in your inner world?

4) *Acceptance*

What do you easily accept that once upon a time you might have hated and rejected?

What do you accept now that makes life go more smoothly?

[Make sure that your referent for acceptance is not resignation or condoning.]

Menu list: Do you accept taking out the garbage, driving in rush hour traffic, a rainy day, etc.?

How is it to just acknowledge what *is*?

Are you willing to accept whatever is in a friendly way?

When you elicit this simple feeling of acceptance and feel it gently in your body, where do you want to put this in your crucible place? How do you represent it so that when you go there you "know" that this resource is there in your inner world? What would be, for you, a good and vivid symbol of acceptance? Perhaps some open hands, or a mailbox, or a wheelbarrow.

5) *Appreciation — Recognizing Positive Intention*

What do you appreciate? What pleasures and delights enable you to melt with appreciation?

What do you appreciate about this experience?

What could you appreciate about it?

Are you even now *melting in appreciation* as you think about that thing?

Again, when you get this feeling, where do you want to put this in your crucible place? How do you represent it so that when you go there you "know" that this resource is there in your inner world? Perhaps a beautiful flower in full bloom, an overview where you can watch a sunset, or a picnic blanket under a big oak tree.

6) Ruthless Honesty for truth-telling — *Authenticity, Speaking and Living the Truth*

Have you ever just said what *is* without judgment, accusation, or attack?

> *Menu list:* Asking for something on a menu at a restaurant, a little child commenting on what he or she sees.

What would that be like if you didn't speak the truth?

Do you have anything to fear from what *is,* from reality, from the truth?

Are you willing to become a friend to reality and be honest about it?

Do you need any self-delusion?

If truth or reality sets us free, especially free from delusions and defenses, what do you need to believe to increase your honesty and truth-speaking?

As you call forth this truth-speaking sense, where do you want to put this in your crucible place? How do you represent it so that when you go there you "know" that this resource is there in your inner world? What would effectively symbolize truth, truth-telling, and/or honesty for you? A special place where the sun shines in brightly in the morning, a round-table like King Arthur's, or a throne of truth?

7) *Ownership and Responsibility*

What is an experience of being responsible that for you has been positive, exciting, and that brought out your very best?

How fully do you feel your mental, emotional, verbal, and behavioral powers to respond to whatever happens?

What do you own that you "know" with every fiber of your being?

How do you experience the feeling or sense of ownership?

As you elicit this sense of the-power-to-respond level of ownership, where do you want to put this in your crucible place? How do you represent it so that when you go there you "know" that this resource is there in your inner world? What would be a great symbol of response-ability or ownership? Perhaps an overview that gives you a panoramic view, a waterfall that generates tremendous power, or a geyser shutting into the sky.

8) The Peak Experience of Love, Joy, Ecstasy, Humor that gives a sense of Vitality Transcendence.

Have you ever just simply and purely loved something with no agenda of your own?

When have you extended yourself for the benefit or welfare of another?

Or when have you experienced a sense of benevolent good will?

When you think about something that you have fallen in love with, what is that like?

As you elicit these feelings, just notice how you code and recognize this in your body.

What is the sense of "Eureka!" like for you?

How do you experience a sudden or even shocking realization of delight, when you are "surprised by joy?"

As you elicit this sense of pure joy and ecstasy, what best represents this for you? A bubbling pool of water, an opening of the heavens, or a rush of love throughout your body and all around you? Do you now have a gorgeous Crucible?

9) Solidify these traits into your Crucible

Take a moment now to be fully present in your crucible place and as you do—just welcome in all of these rich resources as states and frames of mind as I mention them. And as you allow all of these elements in, and represent them in this special space where you can be fully you, and the symbols for each, notice what happens.

What is it like to see the world through the frames of witnessing, accepting, appreciating, an honesty that is ruthlessly truthful, and the ownership of your responses? And when all of these come together is there any emergent sense of beingness or love or joy?

What is this experience as a whole like for you? When you are fully into your Crucible sacred space, what state are you in?

How would you like to anchor it so that you can trigger it at will?

[Anchor the gestalt state of the Crucible using your gestures and posture.]

10) Future pace these resource frames and confirm it.

Imagine fully and completely moving into your tomorrows with these frames of unconditional esteem, witnessing, acceptance, appreciation, and ruthless honesty regarding your needs, emotions, and experiences—are you fully aligned with this?

Does any part of you object to letting this operate as your orientation style?

If so, recycle back to adding in the sufficient resources that you need.
Are there any other resources that you need? [Joy, humor, relaxation, excitement, focus, discipline, etc.]
Would you like this to be how you move through the world?
Are you willing to make this your orientation?
Would this empower you as a person?
Would it enhance your life?
How does it feel to say, "This is my personal Crucible space that enables me to unlearn old responses and to learn new adaptations, and to create changes for next-level transformations!"?

#2 The Crucible Transformation Pattern
If you have built a Crucible space, you are now ready to use the *Crucible* pattern to unleash your highest and best. Are you ready now to *encounter* yourself with your reality, your strengths, weaknesses, possibilities, potentials, responsibilities, choices, needs, emotions, etc.? Are you ready to unlearn things that interfere or sabotage your self-actualization?

As you facilitate this pattern, access your own Crucible elements to create the space for the other person. Continually ask the person, "Are you still in the Crucible?"

As the person experiences thoughts and emotions, simply follow him or her there and ask, "What are you aware of?" "Is that your truth?" "Have you spoken that truth honestly to yourself?" The person could, however, immediately jump to appreciation and tell you the value of the thing. If so, follow him or her there. "And as you notice that value, is that a truth to speak to yourself?" A key to using this pattern effectively is to *follow the person*. Another key is to *direct the process to the various elements* so that they work on the whatever is brought into the Crucible. Before ending, check that the dance has encountered each crucible element.

The Pattern:
1) Identify the interference or problem to the person's self-actualization.
What interferes with your unleashing? What needs to be dealt with?
What will you take into the Crucible to melt down and give a new form and expression?
What does that mean to you?
Okay, so that's what you'd like to take in and encounter for a transformation?

2) Access your crucible space and refresh it.

As you re-access the space of your Crucible, what is the metaphor that you use to convey the sense of safety, witnessing, accepting, appreciating, and truth-telling?
How much are you in the place of witnessing acceptance?
How much are you in the place of embracing the rawness of truth?
What do you need to do to fully access your Crucible?
What do you want to be unleashed *from* and unleashed *to*?

Pre-Encounter Preparation

3) Witnessing it — *explore your matrix of meanings about the interference*.

As you notice what it is, what do you think about it? Where do you go?
Where does your brain take you? What does it mean to you? [Facilitate the person to climb the meaning ladder, the ladder of inference and interpretation.]
As you get a body sense of it, just be with it. What is it like?
How is it to just witness this? How cleanly are you just witnessing it?
Are there any cognitive distortions in it? Which ones have you found?

4) Explore with Acceptance.

As you accept what you are witnessing, what happens?
As you just welcome it in... As you just breathe it in ... and let it be ... noticing it.
How easily are you just acknowledging and accepting it?
Do you now have permission to just acknowledge that this exists or did exist?
Do you have permission for this? Check your permission level:
> Go inside, quiet yourself and say, "I give myself permission to feel X." Upon doing this, notice your internal responses. What would happen if you did accept or experience this negative emotion? How well does that settle inside? What objections, if any, may arise to this?

What resources would you need to access in order to more fully accept this?
> "It's just an emotion."

What other resources would support you?
Do you need to give yourself more permission? How does that settle? How many more times will you need to give yourself

permission so it settles well?

[Troubleshooting with Permission:
> As you quiet yourself, take a moment, perhaps to close your eyes and say within your mind, "I give myself permission to just accept whatever I find."
> Notice any internal responses that might arise as you say this.
> How well does that settle inside? What objections, if any, arise to this?
> What resources would you need to access in order to more fully accept this?
> What reframe of meaning would you like to add to this experience?
> Have you given yourself permission congruently with a strong and resourceful voice so that it reframes the objections? How does that settle inside?
> Examples:
>> "I give myself permission to feel anger because it allows me to recognize things that violate my values and to take appropriate action early."
>> "I give myself permission to feel tender emotions because it makes me more fully human."]

The Encounter of reality and truth
5) *Explore with honesty — ruthless honesty.*
> What are you now aware of?
> Given this, what do you realize?
> Is that the truth? Really?
> Do you absolutely know that it is true? Is it always true?
> Is it true or just familiar and so you feel comfortable with it?
> What truth do you need to tell yourself?
> Is this a truth that you need to speak to yourself?
> What is the reality here that you have not yet seen?
> Is there anything else nudging you in the back of your mind?
> Is there anyone else that you need to speak this to?
> As you now fully feel your truth-speaking ability, consider this specific unleashing of your potentials from something and to something, how is that?

6) *Explore with Appreciation.*
> What can you appreciate about this? What value can you find in it?

What positive intention?
What rich meanings can you give to this?
Feeling this appreciation, what new potentials will this enable you to unleash?
As you access appreciation fully and apply it to all your gifts, aptitudes, strengths, etc., what happens? Where are you now?

7) Take responsibility to speak, own, and do this truth.
What is your decision? What will you decide or choose?
What will you now *do* about this truth?
What actions will this truth now enable you to take?
What will you choose to think, feel, or say?
What response will you now make when X happens?
Do you own this truth? Are you ready to be responsible for it and to it?
Do you need to make an explicit decision to do that?
How much ownership have you already taken about this?
How much more to take?
Do you have full permission to *own* your life, your meanings, emotions, powers, etc.?
How will you handle your excuses?
What will you do about the symptoms?
Now fully feel your ownership, consider this specific unleashing of your potentials from something and to something, how is that?

[Think of all of these elements like dance steps— movements of mind, emotion, and body that you can use and experience. As you are with whatever is brought into the Crucible, just dance with it. Move to this or that resource, notice what happens, and then move to another. There's no right or wrong way. As a facilitator you'll develop your intuitions about this as you keep working with the pattern. Happy dancing!]

Post Encounter Responses
8) Love
What do you now love? What now excites you about your life?
So what's happening? Where are you now?
What are you now able to fall in love with?
Are there any new excitements or passions that have emerged?
What passion have you recovered or new passions have arisen?
If you were to look around and see if you can detect any emerging joy, ecstasy, peak experience— what are you aware of?

9) Consolidate and Integrate.

So, where are you now? What's happened in this process?
What new resources do you now have or that are emerging?
How has X been transformed? Is it an interference any longer?
What transformations are occurring?
What new ways of thinking and feeling and being are emerging for you?
What new choices will you be making because of this?
What have you been unleashed from and unleashed to?

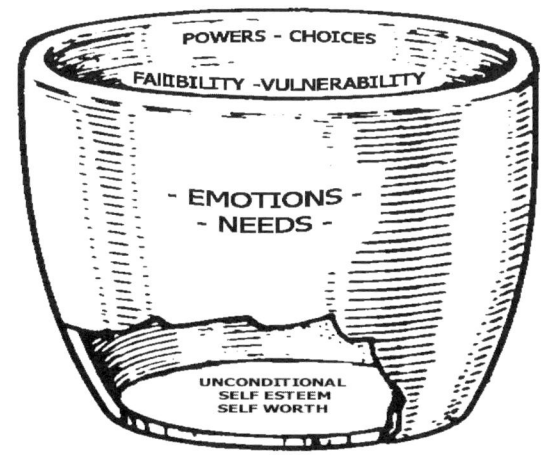

Recovering Previous Unrecognized Crucibles Pattern

Given that there are conditions that make an experience *a crucible for change,* you can now use these as stages of a Crucible experience and begin to use these questions to explore past experiences that you could have used for a transformation. How many Crucible experiences have you been through and yet you did not recognize them as such? When you went through these experiences, you probably passively suffered various negative emotions and drew lots of false and even damaging conclusions. Well, as "It is never too late to have a happy childhood," it is also never too late to use your Crucible experiences for transformative renewal.

The following questions are designed to call forth crucible experiences that you have but didn't recognize and didn't use for transformation. As the questions recover these experiences, you can then take them into the Crucible and use them productively.

1) Heat:

> Has an experience activated intense energy (emotionally, mentally) within you?
> What experience calls upon you, or has called on you, to respond?
> What experience demands something of you? What does it demand?
> What experience puts you under immense pressure?
> What is, or was, that pressure?
> What was, or is, at stake in that experience? What was at risk?
> What kind of energy is or was activated— mental, emotional, a drive?
> How are or were you challenged? Challenged to what?
> How are or were you tested, put to the test?

2) Time-Space:

> Did you stay with the experience for a sufficient time?
> How are you being held in that experience?
> How long has it held you there? Or, how long were you held in it?
> What ways are you, or did you, use to try to escape it?
> How did you try to defend against it?
> What prevents you from escaping?
> What is breaking (or broke) through all of your defenses?
> What forces the encounter?
> What is the fierce conversation that you are now ready to have?
> Is that conversation just within yourself or with someone else?

3) Ownership of Meaning:

> Did you use the experience for personal transformation?
> Did you let the experience evoke, elicit, and provoke inner change in you?
> What and how did you change or do you need to change?
> How were you molded by the experience?
> What dream emerged through the experience?
> What dream are you now actualizing given that experience?
> What decision did you make or do you need to make?
> How did the experience reveal or develop your character?
> What meanings did you release?
> What meanings did you create?

Crucible Coaching
Ideally, it is best to find someone that you trust to facilitate the process of building up the sacred space of your dynamic Crucible. Do you have someone who will do that? Who could you find to do that?

The three specific patterns in this chapter gives you a way to systematically use the principles and elements of the Crucible so you can manage the transformative powers within the Crucible to unlearn an old response and unleash new potentials for your full development. You now know that each element is a resource for change, for growth, and for developing more ego-strength as you face and cope with reality. Each is also a healthy change mechanism for both remedial and generative change.

> So take time this week to use the first pattern to create your inner Crucible Space. And when you have done that to your satisfaction, then use the second pattern to take something that needs changing into your Crucible.
>
> If after the reading and practicing, you are still unsure about how to use these patterns, consult with a professional Meta-Coach. Then you'll have a professional who can guide you through the process and once you learn it, then you'll be able to easily use the patterns with yourself. [www.meta-coachingfoundation.org]

Chapter 15

THE CRUCIBLE CONVERSATION

The Fierce Center at the Heart of Things

A human Crucible is preeminently a place for a conversation— a very special and fierce conversation. There you, or another, encounters a truth, a meaning, responsibility, an appreciation in a dialogue of openness and transparency. It is a conversation that confronts a reality in order that you experience a transformation. Given that, *how* do you carry out this kind of fierce conversation in the Crucible? In the previous chapters you have had a front row seat as you've read some case studies of some fierce conversations. And more are to come.

The Fierce Conversation[1]
First, I'll describe what it is *not*. A "fierce" conversation does *not* involve attacking or being attacked. It is not being aggressive, ugly, mean, cruel, or uncaring. It is none of those things, not at all. The reason we say that it is *fierce* is because it "gets to the heart of things" without cover-ups, roles, personas, masks, and defenses. It is fierce because it cuts through cover-ups and enables you to come face-to-face with truth, with raw reality, and doing that turns up the heat creating emotional intensity. In a fierce conversation you speak the truth regarding what *is* without needing to be politically correct or conventionally polite—these are the factors that typically prevent you from dealing with what's real and actual. No more spin. No more shallow and false "positive thinking." You explore and discuss the brute facts of the case.

Because the fierceness is not in being hard, harsh, mean, or cruel, the fierceness is not in style. *The fierceness is in the context of speaking truth, meaning, and responsibility.* Normally, when you confront or are confronted, there are strong intense emotions. Don't you find that to be the case? The fierceness is in *being real* because it enables you to experience reality in a more direct and raw form. It is fierce because you are not let off the hook, you have to face the mirror of your reflections.

There's a verse in the Bible describes that the quality of this Crucible conversation. The verse says that to reach maturity we have to set aside cunning, crafty deceitfulness and *speak the truth in love* (Ephesians 4:15). That states precisely and succinctly the key idea here. You speak truth with love, with compassion for yourself and others so that you are frankly honest. As you now confront the brute facts of the case without caving in or reacting in defensiveness. After all, you don't need to be afraid of reality or to make yourself an enemy to it.

Within the encounter group movement of the 1960s and 1970s there was a focus on "the truth," on being real, and on giving up all pretenses, and everything the contributes to self-deception. Their focus, as far as that goes, was good. The way they went about it was not. It was generally too rough and therefore failed to provide the safety that's needed. It was as strong on honesty as it was weak on love.

This ability to look reality in the face without falling apart also expresses at its best what we mean by "ego-strength." It takes a strong sense of self (*ego* as in "I" or "me") to fearlessly face reality with a solution-focus orientation. Now you can hold a fierce conversation that can use the power of acceptance to *honestly* face and deal with reality as you find it rather than how you wish it would be. A fierce conversation is not a debate. It is not an argument. That's because the confrontation is with truth, not the other person, it is with what is real and actual—finding it and facing it for whatever it is.

Yet here's the funny part of this— while truth sets us free from lies and deceptions, we all also seem to be afraid of it. It is our best guide and frame in coping with things, and yet so scary. How can that be? What's so scary about truth?

One of the most fearful things about truth is that truth *exposes*. It reveals what is. Like a mirror that simply reflects back what comes into its presence— truth shows us what is. And sometimes, well a lot of the time, we don't really want to see what is. And if you don't want to see what is, then truth becomes dangerous to your peace of mind, your perceptive, your awareness, and your sense of self. It's going to rock your world. And this begins the downward spiral of developing a bad relationship to truth. Scott Peck would say that this is the process by which a person can become one of the "people of the lie."

Another scary thing about truth is that as truth exposes, *truth also challenges you to change.* This is the glory of every mirror. You look in a mirror, and if you see something that doesn't fit for your self-image, that doesn't measure up to your mental map of how you want to present yourself, and the mirror activates you to do something, to make an adjustment.

Truth has a similar effect on us. That's why simply saying a truth aloud introduces change. This is true even if "the truth" is a perceived truth that you'll ultimately discover is false. There's a cleansing effect in speaking the truth as best as you know it at this moment. Doing that sets in motion the energy to act. That which is true engenders action— response. That's why any and every totalitarian, repressive regime finds "freedom of speech" so threatening and dangerous to their rule. So small and large dictators alike are always seeking to suppress any opinion that differs. They know that danger arises when someone speaks out.

So the challenge is to "speak the truth in love." Love enables you to handle the exposure of truth. So adapt the eyes of love so that as you face yourself authentically or invite someone else to have a fierce conversation, love bathes the atmosphere and sets the frame for the encounter.

The Fierceness of the Crucible
Truth is the fierceness of the Crucible. Truth's nature to expose and challenge induces intensity. If into it you then pour the hot sizzling stuff of your human emotions and fallibility, your fears and angers, your hopes and dreams, your loves and excitements, an intensity will arise in the Crucible. Then from out of the human crucible of acceptance, appreciation, and brute honesty comes power, a raw power that can feel dangerous and even threatening. This invites transformation and renewal.

In all of this I've been speaking metaphorically, so what is this all about? And how can you handle the intensity and fierceness of the Crucible? The fierceness is that of reality itself. It is facing whatever *is* on its own terms. You are then empowered to face the raw and brutal facts regardless of your likes, preferences, optimism, beliefs, etc. this is the fierceness of truth.

That's why the human version of a Crucible involves *getting to the*

> *heart of things, holding a space for being with truth, for facing reality as it is, and for holding a fierce existential conversation about all of this.*

It's not often that we experience that kind of conversation. In fact, most of us spend our lives avoiding such. We dissemble, placate, put approval and conventionality above truth, and use all kinds of defense mechanisms. We creatively invent all kinds of excuses. Yet when we do have such a conversation, the experience of a fierce conversation begins an unleashing of potentials. That's because, in the words of Susan Scott, in a fierce conversation "we come out from behind ourselves into the open to be present, open, vulnerable, real," and then we begin to courageously interrogate reality.

In *Coaching Conversations*, I wrote the following about this under the section entitled, "Conversing in the Crucible:"[1]
> "In fierce conversations, we go for the heart of a matter. We relentlessly pursue an experience to understand it and to create space for transformation. Yet doing so we hold the clients' emotions and intense inner experience in the crucible of our commitment to his or her development and we do so with compassion and gentleness, all the while firmly not letting it go. Doing this creates a containment for the client—a place where it is safe to explore." (2004, p. 176)

Holding the clients' truth, emotion, frames, awareness, and experience, as in a Crucible, allows you to have fierce conversations and get to the heart of things. Of course, this requires moral courage, clarity about what you're working and dealing with, and skill for how to converse with a firm gentleness or gentle firmness.

Now in the end, all that you are dealing with is human stuff—just human stuff of thoughts, emotions, sensations in the body, physiology, ideas, beliefs, memories, and imaginations. *In the end all you are dealing with are just frames.* There are nothing more. There are nothing to fear. There are no aliens or demons inside ready to pop out. There's just strong, intense thoughts and emotions that may or may not be accurate to the truth of the situation. So fully embracing the humanness, you can explore it. Again from *Coaching Conversations:*
> "There is another premise that's critical for conversing in the crucible. *It is the frame that the person is never the problem.* The problem is only and always the *frames* that the person is operating in and sometimes (but much less often) the experience is a problem.

> But not the person. The person is doing the best he or she can given those experiences within those frames. When the frames change, the experience will be transformed." (2004, p. 177)

When you engage in fierce conversations you chase down the frames that are creating the distress and flush them out. What is the incredible magic at that point that makes this happen? The secret: *You can't change what we're not aware of.* No wonder awareness is the first step in making changes. In fact, there are times when the mere process of becoming aware of your frames changes them. Sometimes, *awareness per se is curative.* Some changes occur automatically and organically with awareness. When that happens, we say:

> "Oh that's what I've been doing! Oh, that's where that comes from. That's ridiculous! No more of that!"

What makes the fierce conversation safe so you can endure it is the support of the coach, or the person (even if it is yourself) who is holding the higher frames of change, transformation, possibility, opportunity, generating better responses, becoming more skilled, etc. This is what enables the person to stay in the Crucible while facing the inner dragons.[2] In the process, the client learns how to do the same for him or herself.

So in the end, there are several challenges in having a fierce conversation. There is the challenge of staying focused, being in the moment with the client, asking clear and powerful questions, holding the higher frames, holding the client's purposes and outcomes, and modeling the authenticity that we want to evoke.

The Quality of Fierceness

What makes the conversation fierce? What can make you feel like you are sitting in a hot chair? The following are the key factors in the fierceness of the conversation:

1) A content of truth: Your truth, reality, and the brute honesty of speaking what you know at this time.

2) The constraint of holding: You or another person has to be strong enough and focused enough and persistent enough to keep holding the space. You cannot let it go. You must keep coming back to the subject. And not let someone off the hook. Do that and you sell themselves short.

3) The action of acting on and living truth: What will you do? Not just think about, or talk about, or conceptualize, but what will you do? What difference will it make? How will it change things for you?

4) The meanings that have been created: What meaning will you give to a given event or experience? Meaning is what lies at the heart of things. The quality of your meanings is the quality of your life.

5) The existential nature of human life: Questions of existence: who are you? Why are you here? What are you up to? What's important? How should you live? What about your fallibility? Your mortality? Who do you want to become?

Sweating Out the Heat
When I facilitated Ian to face his truths in the Crucible, he began sweaty profusely. Literally. I was actually shocked by how much he sweated. It began when I asked him a simple question, "Are you dismissing this event or truly forgiving him for what he did?"

Wherever his mind took him at that moment, he was in a place of encounter — encountering himself and his response.
    "I just want to drop it. Forget it."

"Okay, so that's your truth at this minute? [Head nodded yes.] Okay, so in dropping it, are you just wiping it away without facing whatever you need to face in yourself or are you truly dropping it because you have faced yourself and made whatever adjustments you needed to make?" Now the sweat really began rolling.
    [Long pause.] "I guess I have not really faced myself. I just wanted to drop it —forget it."

"You've said that several times, yet forgetting is an unconscious process, something that naturally happens when you have truly faced yourself and forgiven. Is this now your truth—that you have not faced yourself?"
    "Yes. I haven't faced myself."

"Are you now ready to? ["Yes"] Okay, so as you bring into the Crucible this past event ... remembering the problem is never you, but always your frames, the ideas that you were acting out... just *be with that awareness*... and allowing yourself to *just witness* that younger you – just witness with a sense of acceptance of what is— *recognizing your unconditional value* as a human being ... go ahead now and face yourself. ... What do you need to face about yourself in this situation? *What is your truth* that's been so scary to face before now?"

>[Sniffing.] "That I wanted him to accept me for myself. I looked up to him more as a father than a partner in our business. But he didn't. He couldn't."

"And your truth?"

>"That I made myself too needy, too dependent, that I pushed him away and made myself despicable in his sight with my attitude and actions. He said I was co-dependent and I hated him for saying that."

"And the frame that drove all of that?"

>"The frame? Ah, that I was treating myself as needy, that I was not good enough. I was wanting him to do the valuing, to value me."

"And when you face that within the context of your own unconditional self-esteem?

>"Well, it was just my ignorance that did all of that."

And your responsibility today?
>To esteem myself.

And will you esteem yourself?
>"Yes. Definitely!"

Crucible Coaching

In your notebook, *My Transformative Life,* devote a page with the title "Love and Truth."

>Divide the page into two columns with *Love* and *Truth* as the headings of each column. If you are now ready to have some fierce conversations with yourself, then fill in statements of love for yourself or another to set the atmosphere. Then write in the *truth* that needs to be said.

>Once you get used to facing your own truths and being ruthlessly honest with yourself, then you'll be able to facilitate fierce conversations with others. What will be the first fierce conversation that you'll have with yourself this week? When and where will you hold that conversation?

>"Truth Conversations Needed" can be another page in your notebook. Here you can make a list of all of the places in life where there is dishonesty, cover-ups, lying promotions that deceive,

hypocrisy, immorality, corruption, dehumanization, anything that undermines the truth. Whenever you encounter one of these, write down the context, person, place, and the content of what was said. This will train you to be able to see reality more clearly and not be deceived by untruths.

End of Chapter References
1. Susan Scott, *The Fierce Conversation* (2002).

2. "Dragons" metaphor, see *Dragon Slaying* (2000).

Chapter 16

COACHING
AND THE CRUCIBLE

Because the Crucible Model is designed for breakthrough transformations for unlearning and new learnings in service of actualizing your highest and best, *the Crucible is a Coaching model par excellence.* Obviously, if I didn't believe that, I would not have put this book in the Meta-Coaching series. Yet, how do you coach it? How do you use the model in an actual coaching session with a client?

Being the Crucible
First of all and most important—be a Crucible for your client. Like Mahatma Gandhi famous statement, "Be the change that you want to create," so with the Crucible.

> *Mentally, emotionally, and inter-personally be the Crucible for your client.*

How? Easy, first unconditionally value and believe in the client. Before you elicit the client's own belief and value in self, you set the pace, you go first. *With unconditional value*—look at, speak with, and engage your client. Start with respectful honor that entails no conditions. Set your perspective to see your client as a sacred and valuable human being and that he or she needs nothing else to be respected and honored.

Act and speak from the premise that, for you, there is no question about the client's value. One characteristic of every great coach that I've interviewed as an expert coach is that the coach believes in the client much more than the client believes in him or herself. The coach sees value, sacrilizes the client, and operates as if that is just a given, a fact. So, how much do you believe in your clients? How much more could you develop your belief in the potentials and possibilities of your clients?

Next, as a coach, *witness whatever you find and observe in the client.* Just witness it. Just observe and then like a mirror, simply reflect it back. Reflect it back with no judgment, no evaluation, no commitment to it being good or bad, just that "I noticed this or that." Be the observation of a clean mirror and model non-judgmental noticing.

Next, *accept and acknowledge whatever you observe.* Welcome it. Embrace it. And do this in a matter-of-fact way. It's usually not something great or even good or even desirable. But if it is there, if it is a fact and condition in the client's life, then acknowledge it. Don't fight it, resist it, try to change it — not at this point. Just accept it. Be the acceptance that the client may not have been able to be, until now.

With these three coaching responses, you have created *in yourself* the safety that operates as that which contains the Crucible. Now you are ready to enter into the furnace of truth where you can welcome the client's heat. So speak the client's truth. Put his or her truth into words. Utter them. Say the unsayable. Express what has never been said before. Take the hushed whispers and the silent internal dialogue and say it aloud. Let the truth be spoken within the context of acceptance, witnessing, and unconditional positive value. Having done that, now you can ask:
>"Is this a truth you want to live? Is there any higher truth than this? If so, what? How are you doing to live this truth? What will you do with this truth? So what?"

If truth is to be lived, then invite the client to live it. If truth sets us free, then we need to speak the truth, hear the truth, live in the space where the truth can be brought out into the open. And that's precisely what you can do here.

Coaching the Crucible involves appreciating the value in the truth. So you go first. Speak the value, point to the value, facilitate the seeing and recognizing of value in the truth. Now you are framing and reframing— presenting the truth in a new light, a light the client hasn't seen. Ask about that. What would seeing things from X perspective do for you? How would that change your life?

Finally, it's time to recognize or evoke a tremendous rush of vitality and joy in order to consciously celebrate the transformations. Here you are priming the pump for the experiencing of a peak experience so the client can begin to allow those special moments to arise and to notice them. So as you began with value— unconditional value for the person, you now close the loop with value for the experience, for life, for insights.

Invite the Crucible Elements as Resources
Being a Crucible is first and most important, yet it is not the only thing you can do in using the Crucible as a model in your coaching. You can also take each and every element and present them to your client as resources. You can turn each of these qualities into a question for exploration.

> How well do you distinguish yourself and your worth from what you do? What decision do you need to make to unconditionally value yourself from this day forward?
> Are you ready to be as kind and gentle with yourself as you are with others? To accept what you can't change?
> If you're convinced that a judgmental attitude doesn't help, are you ready to release all judgment and just witness reality for what it is? To what extent do you know that it is truth that will set you free? Do you know that? Do you know that even small doses of dishonesty work like a poison within?
> How robust is the idea of being "a responsible person" for you? Does it attract you?
> Are you ready to live your life "melting in appreciation" every day? Have you ever looked at life, or others, or some event, or yourself with a sacred perceptive?

Simply bringing up the elements of the Crucible and asking questions about them enables you to coach them, to bring them into the coaching conversation. Each element is a change dynamic in its own right. That is, each of the elements of the Crucible are dynamic principles that facilitate change and learning.

Speak the Truth in Love
Whether you think about Coaching as a profession or using coaching as a methodology for managing, leading, parenting, or collaborating with a friend, coaching today refers to coming out from behind yourself to be real in relation to another. It is about speaking truth as you know it and inviting truth as another person knows it so that the conversation can be real and authentic. And that empowers you to get to the heart of things with loving boldness. It enables you to cut-through defenses, roles, and personas to get

to what really matters.

In Meta-Coaching we describe this kind of fierce and powerful conversation as *a transformational conversation* that's designed to unleash potentials and free a person to become all that he or she can become. It is a conversation like none other— real, earnest, intentional, and highly focused. It is not a wimpy conversation that dances around the truth and that plays nice at the cost of avoiding reality. It faces reality with a belief that people are tough enough to take it, to rise up to meet the challenges of life.

Coaching that uses the Crucible Model as an essential part of the process means laser-beam listening that enables a person to feel truly attended to. Joseph Pine in *The Experience Economy* describes this kind of listening in these words:

> "The experience of being understood, versus interpreted, is so compelling you can charge admission."

This is sacred listening. It is intense listening that believes that if you listen close enough, the person will hand you both the problem and the solution on a platter. This is the kind of listening that will stop your words, especially your advice and solutions, to provide the space for the person to activate his or her own creativity.

Business leaders and managers are discovering the power of this kind of coaching as a way of tapping into the human capital of their people— their intellectual, creative, personal, interpersonal capital.

So what is the Crucible?
The Crucible is a lot of things —
- *The Crucible is a trance, a hypnotic reality.* It arises as an induction into an imagined place in your mind—a place where you are at your best, and a place where you can easily access the safety for change and the resources for a confrontational encounter.

- *The Crucible is a place of encounter.* As such, it empowers you with the energy and the ego-strength to face what needs to be faced. The encounter in the Crucible is an encounter of truth, authenticity, of love, value, sacredness. It is an encounter of responsibility and ownership.

- *The Crucible is an attitude of respect, acceptance, witnessing, truth-telling, appreciating, and responsibility.*

- *The Crucible is a metaphor that facilitates profound communication.* And the conversation is profound because it allows a person to get to the heart of things to both unlearn what's no longer valid and create new meanings for living more fully.

Appendix A

INDEX
COGNITIVE DISTORTIONS

Mastering Cognitive Distortions

The following list of cognitive distortions come from RET (Rational Emotive Therapy) of Albert Ellis and Aaron Beck. The Meta-Model distinctions come from NLP (*Structure of Magic I and II; Communication Magic*). These distinctions relate to *how a person thinks* and therefore sorts for and processes information. The point here is that the quality of your meaning-making is a function of the quality of your thinking so often it is not *what* you are thinking or the meaning that you are creating but *how* you are thinking and encoding those meanings.

Name of the Distinction	Meta-Model	Healthy Cognitive Processing
1. Over-generalizing	Generalizing	Contextual thinking
2. Judging; Evaluating		Description; sensory-based thinking
3. All-or-nothing thinking	Universal Quantifiers	Both-and; in-between thinking
4. Labeling; Nominalizing	Nominalizing	Reality-testing thinking; denominalizing
5. Thingify-ing	Nominalizing	Process, systems thinking
6. Identifying	Identification	E-prime / dis-identifying thinking
7. Simplifying		Systems thinking
8. Discounting	Deleting	Appreciative thinking
9. Mind-reading	Mind-Reading	Current sensory information
10. Prophesying		Tentative predictive thinking
11. Filtering out; Deleting	Deleting	Perspective / Perspective thinking
12. Blaming		Responsibility thinking
13. Emotionalizing	CEq	Witness thinking or non-emotionalizing
14. Personalizing	Identification	Objective thinking
15. Awfulizing	Pseudo-words	Meta-cognitive thinking
16. Should-ing	Modal Operator	Choice thinking
17. Impossibility thinking Can't-ing	Modal Operator	Possibility thinking

Appendix B

META-COACHING

Meta-Coaching is the form of coaching that comes from the field of Neuro-Semantic NLP and we believe it is the most systematic approach to Coaching in the world. We make that assertion based on having defined "coaching" in terms of seven distinctions and from those distinctions have provided more than seven cutting-edge models to address them. This then enables a licensed Meta-Coach to be able to answer the question:
> *How do you know what to do, when to do it, with whom to do it, how to do it, and why?*

To be able to answer that question a coach has to have a theoretical framework (*the why*) that guides *what* to do, at the right time (*the when*) with distinctions about the personality of the client (*with whom*), and a competency (*the how to do it*). A further distinction which makes Meta-Coaching unique is that it is based explicitly on the kind of psychology that governs how psychologically healthy people develop and transform, *Self-Actualization Psychology*.

Books in the Meta-Coaching Series:
1) *Coaching Change:* Axes of Change Model
2) *Coaching Conversations*
3) *Unleashed:* A Guide to Your Ultimate Self-Actualization
4) *Self-Actualization Psychology*: Bright Side of Human Nature
5) *Achieving Peak Performance*
6) *Unleashing Leadership:* Self-Actualizing Leaders and Companies
7) *The Crucible*: Self-Actualization Change Model
8) *Benchmarking* (due in 2011)

Supplementary Books for Meta-Coaching:
9) *Figuring Out People* (2006): Meta-Programs Model
10) *Secrets of Personal Mastery* (1997): Meta-States Model
11) *The Matrix Model* (2003)

For more about Meta-Coaching, see
www.meta-coaching.org and www.metacoachfoundation.org.

BIBLIOGRAPHY

Allport, Gordon. (1971). *Becoming: Basic considerations for a psychology of personality.* New Haven: Yale University Press.

Assagioli, Roberto. (1965). *Psychosynthesis.* New York: Hobbs, Dorman.

Bandler, Richard; and Grinder, John. (1975, 1976). *The structure of magic, Volumes I and II: A book about language and therapy.* Palo Alto, CA: Science & Behavior Books.

Bateson, Gregory. (1972). *Steps to an ecology of mind.* New York: Ballatine.

Csiksezentmihalyi, Mihaly. (1991). *Flow: The psychology of optimal experience.* New York: Harper & Row.

Fosdick, Harry Emerson. (1943). *On being a real person.* New York: Harper and Brothers, Publishers.

Frankl, Viktor. (1959). *Man's search for meaning.* Boston: Beacon Press.

Gallwey, W. Timothy. (1974). *The Inner Game of Tennis.* NY: Random House.

Gardner, Howard. (1983). *Frames of mind: The theory of multiple intelligences.* NY: BasicBooks.

Gardner, Howard. (1983). *Multiple intelligences: The theory in practice.* NY: BasicBooks.

Glasser, William. (1976). *Positive Addiction.* New York: Harper & Row.

Goleman, Daniel. (1997). *Emotional intelligence: Why it can matter more than IQ.* New York: Bantam Books.

Goleman, Daniel. (2002). *Working with Emotional Intelligence.* London: Bloomsbury.

Hall, L. Michael. (1987). *Motivation: How to be a Positive Force.*

Hall, L. Michael. (2007). *Meta-States: Managing the higher levels of your mind's reflexivity.* Clifton, CO: Neuro-Semantic Publications.

Hall, L. Michael; Bodenhamer, Bob G. (2005). *Sub-Modalities: Going Meta.* Formerly, The structure of Excellence. Clifton, CO: Neuro-Semantic Publications.

Hall, L. Michael. (2000). *Secrets of personal mastery: Advanced techniques for accessing your higher levels of consciousness.* Wales, UK: Crown House Publications.

Hall, L. Michael. (2001). *Communication Magic.* Wales, UK: Crown House Publications.

Hall, L. Michael; Duval, Michelle. (2004). *Coaching Conversations:* Robust Conversations that Coach for Excellence. Clifton, CO: Neuro-Semantic Publications.

James, William. (1890). *Principles of psychology.* Vol. 1. New York: Henry Holt Co.

Jourard, Sydney. (1971). *The Transparent Self.* NY: Van Nostrand Reinhold.

Korzybski, Alfred. (1933/ 1994). *Science and sanity: An introduction to non-Aristotelian systems and general semantics,* (5th. ed.). Lakeville, CN: International Non-Aristotelian Library Publishing Co.

Kuhn, Thomas S. (1970). *The structure of scientific revolutions* (2nd ed.). Chicago: University of Chicago Press.

Lakoff, George; Johnson, Mark. (1980). *Metaphors we live by.* Chicago, IL: The University of Chicago Press.

Maslow, Abraham H. (1943). "A Theory of Human Motivation," *Psychological Review*, L, pp. 370-396. American Psychological Association.

Maslow, Abraham. (1970). *Motivation and Personality.* (2nd ed.). New York: Harper & Row.

Maslow, Abraham. (1968). *Toward a Psychology of Being.* New York: Van Nostrand.

Maslow, Abraham. (1953, 1971). *The Farther Reaches of Human Nature.* New York: Viking.

May, Rollo. (1969). *Love and Will.* New York: Norton.

May, Rollo. (1961). *Existential Psychology.* New York: Random House.

Perls. Fritz. (1973). *The gestalt approach and eyewitness to therapy.* Palo Alto: Science and Behavior books.

Polkinghorne, Donald. (1983). *Methodology for Human Sciences.* Albany N: State University of New York Press.

Rogers, Carl R. (1951). *Client-centered therapy.* Boston: Houghton Mifflin.

Rogers, Carl R. (1972). *On Becoming a Person.* Boston: Houghton Mifflin.

Satir, Virginia. (1972). *Peoplemaking.* Palo Alto, CA: Science and Behavior Books.

Seligman, Martin E.P; Csiksezentmihalyi, Mihaly. (2000, Jan.). <u>Positive Psychology: An Introduction.</u> American Psychologist, American Psychological Association, Inc.

Tournier, Paul. (1957). *The meaning of persons.* New York: Perennial Library, Harper and Row Publishers.

Wachowski, Larry; Wachowski, Andy. (2000). Screenplay: *The art of the matrix.* New York: Village Roadshow Films.

INDEX

Acceptance: 26, 31, 70, 81-82, 91, chapter 9 (109-119), 172, 176, 191
    Pattern: 115-117, 118
Alchemy: 37
Appreciation: 27, 31, 71, 86, 92, chapter 11 (137-146), 172, 178.
Authenticity: 26, 49, 81, 129.
Awareness: 97-100.

Change: chapter 2 (19-28), 39, chapter 14 (170-185), 186, 190.
   Kinds and Dimensions: 20
   Axes of Change: 22-24, 77
Choice: 12
Coaching: 2, chapter 16 (190-195).
Cognitive Dissonance: 132, 135
Cognitive Unconscious: 136
Cognitive Distortions: 195
Confrontation: 26
Conversation: 37, 71, 94, 103-106, 126, 130-131, 133, chapter 15 (182-189).

Crucible: 29-30, 61.
   Definition: 1,8.
   Elements: 46-53, 192.
   Natural: 69-70, 73-74.
   Stories: 15, 34, 353, 41-43, 65-66, 100-102, 117, 121-124, 130, 134, 140-143, 150-151, 160-161, 187-188.

Defense Mechanisms: 61, 126.
Dichotomizing: 98-99.
Dis-Identifying: 44-46.
Dragon States: 62, 67.

Ego Strength: 38, 43, 90, 126, 183.
Emotions: 50, chapter 5 (55-67).
   EQ: 56.
   Definition: 57.
   Pattern: Meta-Stating Emotions: 62-63.

Encounter: 4, 51, 68.
   Encounter groups: 3, 47-48, 183, 193.
Empathy: 48, 102, 106.
Expectations: 99-100, 116
Fierce: 182-184, 186.
Forgiveness: 114
Frame: See Meaning.
Heat: 75, 180.
Honesty: see Truth.
HPM: Human Potential Movement: 3, 4, 46.
Humor: 114.
Hypnosis: 5, chapter 14 (170-181), 193.
Human Needs: 33, 55-56.
Human Nature: 80.
Instinct: 38.
Introjection: 116.
Jargon Alerts: 17, 20, 21, 22, 98, 138.

Love: 27, 72, chapter 13 (163-168), 178.
Matrix:
   Model: 8, 10, 18
   The Movie: 9-14, 18.
Meaning: 60, 76, 127-128, 132-133, 138, 143, 145, 164, 185 (frames).
   Explanatory Style: 74

NLP: 102-103, 139.
Neuro-Semantics: 100.
Ownership: 26, 76, 173, 180.

Patterns:
   Meta-Stating Self: 90-94.
   Meta-Stating Acceptance: 115-117, 118.
   Meta-Stating Emotions: 62-63.
   Accessing Appreciation: 143-144.
   Crucible Construction: 170-175.
   Crucible Transformation: 175-

179.
    Recovering Unrecognized Crucibles: 179-180.
Peak Experiences: 27, 72, 164-168, 174.
Permission: 100-102.
Perceptual Positions: 102-103.
Relationship: 158-159.
Responsibility: 72, chapter 12 (147-162), 173, 178.
  Responsibility to/for: 153-160.
sacrilize: 138.
Safety: 70, 191.

Self:
  Self-Actualization: 2, 9, 14, 33, 65, 69, 139, 163-168.
    Self-Discovery: 46.
    Self-Esteem: 83-88.
      Pattern: Meta-Stating Self: 90-94.
    Self-Confidence: 83-88.
    Self-Efficacy: 88-89.

Synonon: 35.
Tested: 13.
Time: 75, 180.
Trance: see Hypnosis.
Truth: 26, 71, chapter 10 (120-135), 173, 177, 183-184, 192.
Unconditional Positive Regard: 25, 48, chapter 7 (80-95), 171.
Unlearning: 39-40, 41-43.
Velveteen Rabbit: 125.
Vitality: 163-168.
Witnessing: 26, chapter 8 (96-108), 172, 176, 191.

Persons:
Bandler, Richard: 99.
Block, Peter: 120.
Brandon, Nathaniel: 147.
Christ, Jesus: 120.
Dunn, Joseph: 109, 113, 116.
Eliot, T.S.: 36.
Freud, Sigmund: 100, 120.
James, William: 59.
Genovese, Kitty: 162.
Gottman, John: 114.
Gandhi, Mahatma: 190.
Frankl, Viktor: 147, 148, 165.
Maslow, Abraham: 3, 14, 29, 30, 35-36, 39, 49-50, 55, 68, 80, 96, 99, 100, 106, 109, 110-111, 120, 127, 137, 147, 153, 159, 163, 164, 165, 167.

Perls, Fritz: 97-98, 121.
Pine, Joseph: 193.
Polkinghorne, Donald: 126.
Rogers, Carl: 3, 47-48, 81, 96, 131.
Schutz, Will: 120, 152.
Walsh, Jim: 25.

AUTHOR

L. Michael Hall, Ph.D. From his studies in many disciplines, from psychology, linguistics, theology, NLP, systems, therapy, etc. Dr. Hall became a *modeler of human excellence and especially of people engaged in self-actualizing activities,* which in turn led to the focus of Neuro-Semantics on "actualizing excellence."

After he studied NLP in 1986, he began using it to model "the highest and best in human experiences." His modeling began from his studies of NLP, then Bateson, Korzybski, and then in his re-discovery of Maslow's original modeling of self-actualizing people. Prior to that Dr. Hall operated a private psychotherapy practice in Colorado, then traveled internationally as a trainer, in 1994 he launched a publishing company, and is now the visionary leader of Neuro-Semantics.

Dr. Hall's first modeling project was on *Resilience* led to the discovery of the Meta-States Model. As a modeler of positive psychological experience, he has modeled numerous experiences and has created many models that now make up the heart of Neuro-Semantics —Meta-States, Matrix Model, the Axes of Change model, Meta-Coach Training system, etc.

1992-1994	Resilience
1992-1996	Reflexivity and *Meta-States* (2008)
1996	Sales, Selling
1995-1996	State Management; Defusing Hotheads
1997-1998	Women in Leadership
1997-1999	Wealth Creation; Inside-Out Wealth
1999-2000	Weight Management and Fitness
2000	Writing Skills
2001	Business Leaders; *Games Business Experts Play* (2002)
2001	Cultures and Cultural Modeling
2001-2009	Coaching for *Meta-Coach Training System*
2003-2004	Change / Transformation; *Coaching Change* (2003)
2003-2009	Self-Actualization processes and psychology
2007-2009	Self-Actualizing Leadership

Dr. Hall has advanced degrees in Biblical language and literature with a focus on Koine Greek and ancient Hebrew; a B.S. in Human Resource Management; M.A. in Clinical Counseling / Psychology; Regis University, and Ph.D. in Cognitive Psychology, Union Institute University.

In working with Richard Bandler he wrote several books for him and then about NLP (*The Spirit of NLP,* 1996; *Becoming a More Ferocious Presenter,* 1996). Upon discovering the Meta-States Model, the *International NLP Trainer's Association* (INLPTA) recognized Dr. Hall for developing "The most significant contribution to the development of the NLP model in 1994/5."

In 1996 Hall and Bodenhamer registered "Neuro-Semantics" and founded *The*

International Society of Neuro-Semantics (ISNS) as a new approach to teaching, training, and using NLP. The objective was to take NLP as a model and field to a higher level in terms of professional ethics. Today Neuro-Semantics is one of the leading disciplines within NLP pioneering many new developments and demonstrating a creativity that characterized NLP when it was new and fresh.

Dr. Hall is known as a prolific writer, having authored 40 books in the field of NLP, many of them best sellers through *Crown House Publishes* (Wales, UK) and many of them translated into numerous languages: German, Dutch, Italian, Spanish, Russian, Japanese, Chinese, Arabic, etc.

www.neurosemantics.com
www.meta-coaching.org
www.self-actualizing.org
www.ns-trainings.com

For Books from
    Neuro-Semantic Publications (NSP)
    P.O. Box 8
    Clifton, CO. 81520—0008 USA
    (970) 523-7877